Women's
VAGINA
UNIVERSITY

A COMPLETE OWNER'S MANUAL
FROM SEX AND PERIODS TO HEALTH AND BODY IMAGE . . .
AND EVERYTHING IN BETWEEN

BY THE EDITORS OF **Women'sHealth**
AND SHEILA CURRY OAKES,
WITH A FOREWORD BY MICHELLE THAM METZ, MD, OB-GYN

RODALE.

This book is intended as a reference volume only, not as a medical manual. The information given here is designed to help you make informed decisions about your health. It is not intended as a substitute for any treatment that may have been prescribed by your doctor. If you suspect that you have a medical problem, we urge you to seek competent medical help.

Copyright © 2018 by Hearst Magazines, Inc.

All rights reserved.
Published in the United States by Rodale Books, an imprint of the Crown Publishing Group, a division of Penguin Random House LLC, New York.
crownpublishing.com
rodalebooks.com

RODALE and the Plant colophon are registered trademarks of Penguin Random House LLC.

WOMEN'S HEALTH is a registered trademark of Hearst Magazines, Inc.

Library of Congress Cataloging-in-Publication Data is available.

ISBN 978-1-63565-175-1
Ebook ISBN 978-1-63565-176-8

Printed in the United States of America

Book design by Jordan Wannemacher
Illustrations by Charlie Layton
Cover design by Amy C. King

10 9 8 7 6 5 4 3 2 1

First Edition

CONTENTS

FOREWORD

It is one of those mornings. I'm running around like a maniacal octopus, reheating rice and black beans for the kids' lunch, cutting up watermelon, and yelling—there is a lot of yelling. I forget to eat breakfast and rush out the door, eyeliner streaked under my left eye, looking a bit more like a wide receiver than a gynecologist. I thank my lucky stars my husband made me that cortado I had to sadly chug instead of savor as I scurry out of the house. Mondays are not always like this, but sometimes the challenges of staying up late to deliver babies *and* deliver organic hot lunches to my kids collide.

Motherhood in all its delicious baby cuddling, babbling first words, and potty success joy is hard. It's damn hard. It has helped me to become a better doctor and human, though. After the birth of my first babe, Maika, I was so fortunate to be able to stay home for 14 weeks to nurse and love her. That period of time in some ways was more challenging than my ob-gyn residency (think 4 years of 30-hour shifts without sleep and well-coiffed, scalpel-wielding women screaming in your face about proper suturing technique). Ob-gyns are trained to deal with hemorrhages, seizures, and ruptured uteruses; no one trained me to strap a 9-pound crying burrito to my chest while cooking dinner and trying to heal from a C-section. To be fair, it helps that crying burritos tend to be supercute. Caring for women, guiding them along their reproductive journey, and delivering their babies came a bit more naturally for me than looking after myself during pregnancy and the breastfeeding years that followed. Boy, was I surprised to find I wasn't more prepared to be a mom myself after so many years of coaching others toward motherhood.

Talks about vaginal lumps and bumps, weird periods, cervical mucus, pain with sex while breastfeeding (yes, that's a thing), and genital warts are just normal parts of my every day. Some of my favorite phrases include "Your uterus is shaped like an upside-down pear" and "The herpes virus has so much stigma attached to it, but it's just a virus; no one gets embarrassed confessing they have had chicken pox, right?" I can honestly say that most of the time those conversations don't feel like work, even though it's actually my job. I strive to be a source of well-curated medical information while still being an open, caring soul. It's incredibly rewarding. From the time I first told my friends that I wanted to be an ob-gyn, it was like the floodgates opened. All the things they had been dying to ask someone, secrets they feared would horrify, embarrass, shame them, suddenly flowed freely. There was a calming relief once the words came tumbling out. I can't tell you how many times a day

I hear, "I have never told anyone this before, but . . ." How over-joyed are these women when I tell them I just treated someone else with the same complaint last week! It's unbelievably com-forting to discover you aren't alone in your abnormal Pap test or urinary dribbles. Feeling a sense of community with all the other newly sexually active women and their recent diagnoses of HPV is kind of reassuring.

I can remember hiding in the produce aisle at ShopRite while my parents paid for my tampons mixed in with a cartload of half-price cabbage and chicken drumsticks, petrified of being associated with those cotton sticks. I felt like a pariah in gym class, having to change those damn things. I mean, this was the reality that 50 percent of my classmates were dealing with, and it was as if we were all standing alone on our solitary islands of period embarrassment. I don't know how my daughter will feel about feminine hygiene products, but I hope by the time she needs them, being open about periods won't be a point of shame. I hope she'll never call me crying from her shower in college because she's confused about contraception and has no one to turn to. I hope she'll know how to talk about female anatomy in a way that is factual and respectful. I hope that she and her peers will have been educated about reproduction with an approach that is far less mysterious and vague than what I learned in eighth-grade health class.

Whenever I think I have discovered a new and impossible patient misunderstanding about the workings of the female body, I am consistently amazed that an even more outrageous anecdote crosses my path. I don't know who perpetuates these myths, but they have somehow managed to withstand time and the Internet! So many women don't know that babies and urine come from different orifices. That sentence has a bit of shock value, but it's a common misconception that I dispel for many first-time moms. I once had a patient swallow condoms thinking that was how they prevented pregnancy. I have discovered entire heads of garlic hidden in patients' vaginas as a naturopathic cure for yeast infections. I have learned more than one culture uses a potato as a makeshift pessary—a sort of a plug placed in the vagina to keep the bladder or uterus from falling down after childbirth (admittedly, I may have explained this term to my husband on one of our first dates. I knew he was a keeper when he didn't run away screaming after this conversation!). A woman in her late forties who had already gone through a full battery of tests for pelvic pain came to me only to discover she was actually 18 weeks pregnant and not, in fact, going through menopause with irritable bowel syndrome. I hope I've been able to handle those confusing moments for patients with grace and compassion. I remind myself to stand in my patients' shoes, with years of old wives' tales flooding their minds and the cultural taboos surrounding our vaginas overpowering their natural instincts. It's been a slow road, but more and more women are taking charge of their reproductive health, and it sure is making my role in the whole process smoother.

It's wonderful that *Women's Health* magazine has a platform and amazing writers to put this information out there in a way that is accessible and, frankly, an open book. I am fortunate to have been asked to work with this team that advocates for women and is even willing to publish this helpful guide with the word "vagina" in big bold letters on the cover!

Empowering women to have a strong voice in their health benefits our society as a whole. There's little to be gained from shrouding the facts of female reproduction in secrecy, as if too precious to be spoken aloud. Sitting beside you on a crowded subway train, maybe the passenger to your right or left once had her uterus swell to the size of watermelon to accommodate a baby, once bled for a month after a miscarriage, once cried herself to sleep fearing she had cervix cancer, once had milk spray from her nipples, once had to stand at the pharmacy counter and say "Plan B" out loud, and she came to me and told me her story. Those stories help other women. Being an ob-gyn has a lot to do with prescribing the right meds to fix your itches and soothe your sore parts, finding you help when the multitasking of new motherhood feels like an overwhelming, tearful burden, but it has a lot to do with storytelling, too. I'm so lucky women trust me enough to tell me theirs.

Michelle Tham Metz, MD

INTRODUCTION

WELCOME TO VAGINA UNIVERSITY!

IT IS WITH GREAT pleasure that we inform you that you have been accepted for admission to Vagina University—welcome! Your SAT or ACT scores don't matter here, but you will find that PMS is a relevant part of the curriculum, and by virtue of owning a vagina, you are have free admission for life. In the time you spend with us, we hope that you will learn more about your body—especially that powerful little organ called the vagina. We would like to clear up any misunderstandings or misinterpretations of the whys and hows of female reproductive health and have some fun learning along the way.

Vagina University was founded by the editors of *Women's Health* magazine and became a section on the Web site Womenshealthmag.com to educate, empower, and inform women. We've written blogs, published articles, and compiled listicles tackling issues like "Your Vagina On Sex" and "Nine Weird Vagina Issues—Solved!"—all the while talking to experts and doctors to keep our advice on the cutting edge. This book takes on all vagina-related issues, questions, and more, digging a little deeper and expanding on the discussions to place the information in context so that you will gain a more complete understanding of your awesome, complex, wonderful vaginal and reproductive self.

Don't worry—it's not at all like a textbook or health class (although we are going to take you on a tour of your lady parts just in case you need a refresher course or if you have never dared to look "down there"). We are going to cover the basics of your anatomy and reveal how all your amazing parts work together. From periods to PMS, from embarrassing itches to health concerns, from hair removal to hormones, we will cover it all.

We'll help you better understand your hormones and why you act, think, and feel the way you do when they are off balance. And your monthly unwelcome visitor? Well, we'll talk about that, too, and how to best manage that situation, perhaps moving away from seeing that time of the month as a "curse" and more of a simple fact of life. Sometimes, if we think of something as dreaded and awful, it becomes dreaded and awful, but maybe we can flip the switch on your period perspective! We'll lift a bit of that stigma and help you sail through that unpleasant stretch with some clever and effective coping mechanisms from pads and tampons, to herbs and yoga, to medications and help from your trusty gynecologist. And if your period is truly troublesome, we hope that some of the information and strategies we provide here can help you not just survive your monthly menace but resolve issues or find ways to reduce the impact of your period on your life so you can live the way the smiling women in tampons commercials do—or as close to it as possible.

To that end, we will share with you warning signs of potential health issues that may seem as if they just come with the menstrual territory but that should really be looked into by a medical professional. We hope to give you information so you can have a much clearer sense of what is typical and establish your own baseline of "normal"—with the caveat that what is "normal" for you might not be "normal" for your best friend—so that you know when you should seek medical care and information. Should you find yourself facing a health issue, we will outline some of the most common diagnoses that women face, explain the symptoms and solutions, and give practical self-help advice so you can better manage a disorder, disease, or infection.

VU is not all about itches and illnesses because—like at every college or university—there is sex! Yes, we are going to talk about gender, sex, sexuality, and sexual identity. We'll cover the mechanics (how to insert slot A into tab B—and variations on that theme), but we'll also talk about how sex isn't only about the mechanics, and that being able to communicate what you want and understand your body and how it responds to stimulation will get you where you want to go: to the Big O. We'll talk about sexual wellness and intimacy, too, and because safer sex is always your best option whenever you hit the sheets—we'll tell you how safer is sexy!

And because we live in the real world, and it can seem that simply being a woman can draw unwelcome attention on the street and in the workplace, we'll cover what can happen, what crosses a line, and your options for coping and making it stop. The Internet will get some attention, too: Because we all spend time online, we'll give you pointers on how to stay safe when you are clicking and swiping all day and all night. We will also cover issues like consent, harassment, and rape as well as how to advocate for yourself and keep yourself safe.

We're looking forward to spending time with you at VU, and we are confident that the knowledge you gain here will serve you well as you bring greater understanding to an important part of your anatomy and empower yourself to take charge of your physical and sexual health and self.

1

ANATOMY 101: VULVA OR VAGINA— DEMYSTIFYING "DOWN THERE"

THERE SEEMS TO BE a taboo about talking about a woman's "lady parts."

When was the last time you heard someone say "vagina" loud and proud? Even when speaking to girlfriends, the v-word, if spoken at all, is often whispered or referred to with some sort of overly cute or silly euphemism. Let's just agree to stop this right now. Culturally, we seem to want to keep our private parts, well, private. But even if you don't ever say the word aloud or prefer to use a nickname, you should know the proper names for your genitals. No worries if you are shy about discussing it—you aren't the only one. Many women don't like to talk about "down there." The thing is, if you ignore a part of your body, never get to know proper terminology, and don't become familiar with its appearance, you are cutting yourself off from important knowledge that can have a significant impact on both your sexual wellness and your overall health.

While you might not want to bust out the vagina/vulva talk in the middle of a business meeting or at the dinner table, it is a good idea to be able to name and claim all aspects of your body—it's actually empowering. Some women become uncomfortable discussing these specific parts of their anatomy, not only in casual conversation with friends but even with their doctors or gynecologists, which doesn't make for a particularly productive appointment. It's bad enough that you are having the conversation while you are concentrating on keeping your behind covered with a paper gown; take back some control of the situation by knowing what's what and where it is and what it's called and what it is for. Understanding the proper names and location of the parts of your genitals also makes good health sense, because if an issue comes up you will be able to give accurate information to your healthcare professional—without whispering or blushing. Well, maybe you will blush, but at least you will be whispering the accurate names of your girl parts. And because you will be speaking the same language, you'll also know just what your doctor is talking about when he or she works with you to resolve any issues.

EXTERNAL ANATOMY

If you, like many women, have been generally referring to the area between your legs as your "vagina," you may be surprised to learn that you have been calling it by the incorrect name. Or the less-than-specific name. It's really common, so don't be embarrassed. Most people call the whole kit and caboodle the vagina, but there is a lot more going on down there.

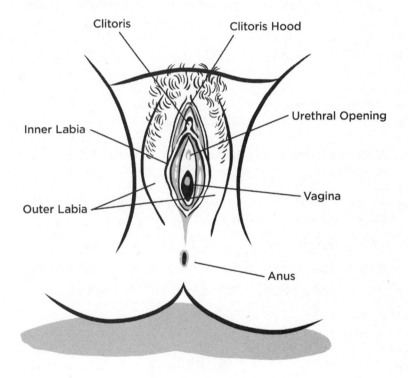

VULVA

What many call the "vagina" is actually the external genitalia, technically called the vulva, and is where the pubic hair grows—unless you've been waxing, shaving, and plucking (more on that later). The vulva is made up of the pubic mound, or mons pubis, which is fatty tissue over the pubic bone, as well as the inner and outer lips—aka labia majora and labia minora.

LABIA MAJORA

The labia majora—sometimes called the outer lips—is the protective layer of fat covered by skin and hair and the most visible part of your vulva. These outer folds help protect your pubic bone when you are having sex. They give a little cushion when you are pushin'.

LABIA MINORA

The more sensitive, thinner, and usually smaller hairless area within the outer lips is called the labia minora, or inner lips. These folds of skin surround and protect the opening to the vagina, the clitoris, and the opening to the urethra. The labia protect the vagina from bacteria, and they also play a significant role in arousal, because hiding at the top of the labia minora, under the clitoral hood, is the infamous clitoris.

CLITORIS

That little love button known as the clitoris takes refuge under a hood because it is so sensitive that it needs to be protected from overstimulation—there are over 8,000 nerve endings in that tiny organ alone, which is twice the amount in a penis. There is more to the clit than meets the eye however: The clitoral glans—the technical term for the visible little nub of the clitoris—is the just the tip of an internal organ that extends in a

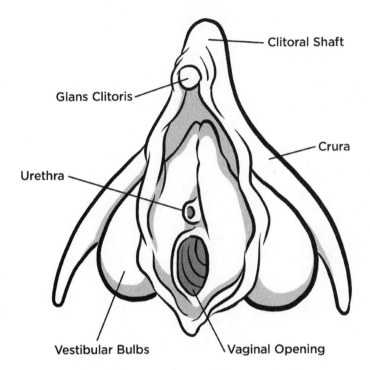

shaft toward the pubic bone, surrounding the vagina, and splits into two legs that are shaped like a wishbone. Composed of erectile tissue—meaning it fills with blood and swells when aroused—this organ contains an additional 15,000 nerve endings, making it the pleasure center in bodies that have them.

LUCKY YOU!

The clitoris is the only part of the human body that has one sole purpose—pleasure!

URETHRA

This tiny opening underneath the clitoris is tough to see, but rest assured that it's there and it's the end of a tiny tube leading from your bladder where urine exits the body.

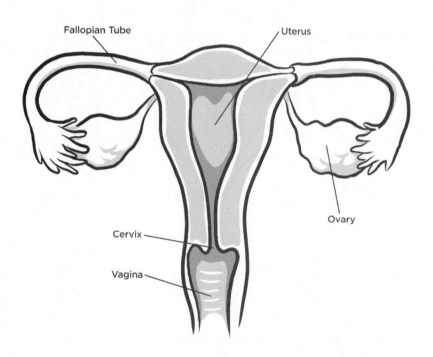

INTERNAL ANATOMY

Although out of sight, parts of your internal anatomy are key players in sex, sexuality, pleasure, satisfaction, and, yes, procreation.

VAGINA

The external anatomy is the gatekeeper, and it protects the internal anatomy, aka the vagina. Your vagina is essentially a tube that is anywhere from approximately 4 to 7 inches long (depending on the woman)—about the length of a tube of lip gloss to the length of a pen. The vagina is very versatile and is involved in sex/sexual activity (it can accommodate penises, fingers, tongues, and sex toys), allows menstrual blood to flow out of the body, and is the canal the baby travels down from the uterus when it is born. The interior walls of the vagina can be a bit lumpy and bumpy because there are folds in the lining that allow the vagina to expand for sex and delivering a baby. The vagina also has nerve endings that respond to stimulation and cause pleasure, just not as many as the vulva or clitoris.

BARTHOLIN'S GLANDS

Found on either side of the lower end of the vaginal opening, Bartholin's glands help lubricate the labia and vagina during sex. The lubrication begins when you are aroused, also known as getting "wet," and is essential in protecting the delicate tissues from injury due to friction from overenthusiastic sex, strenuous exercise, or from those too-tight jeans that look great but don't feel so great.

TILTED UTERUS

Some women have what is known as a tilted uterus, meaning that instead of their uterus looking like the diagrams on the instruction in the tampon boxes, it tilts toward the front or goes straight up. If you are told you have a tilted uterus, it is usually no big deal. The only thing you might notice is that you may have some pain in certain sexual positions (like woman on top) because the penetration may make contact with your tilted uterus. If you experience unusual levels of pain during intercourse, speak with your doctor—only the doc can tell for sure. Ask your gyno at your next appointment to find out if you are one of the 30 percent of women who have a tilted uterus.

G-SPOT

If you were to insert your finger a couple of inches into the opening of your vagina and hook it back toward your front (closer to your belly than your back), you may feel a spongy area that is known as the G-spot—this area can be the source of some mind-blowing orgasms, so it's good to know its location. Long misunderstood, the G-spot is actually the ends of the two wishbone-like ends of the clitoris! We'll be revisiting the G-spot later. Once you know more about it, you will probably want to visit the G-spot more often, too!

CERVIX

At the top of the vaginal canal is the cervix, which is the opening to the uterus. The cervix is responsible for the mucus that
changes during your cycle, and it's the part that your gyno is
swabbing when you get a Pap test. It remains tightly closed and
dilates only to allow menstrual bloodflow and the baby to exit
the uterus when a woman is giving birth.

UTERUS

Flexible and capable of expanding with a baby's growth, going
from the size of your fist to the size of a substantial watermelon,
the uterus—often called the womb—is shaped like an upside-
down pear. Approximately every 30 days or so, the uterus sheds
its lining, and anyone who has a uterus menstruates, unless a
fertilized egg has implanted itself in the uterine lining, meaning the owner of that uterus is pregnant. No periods when you
are pregnant! (More on that in Chapter 2.)

ENDOMETRIUM

The lining of the uterus is tissue called the endometrium. In
some women, the tissue will migrate outside of the uterus
and grow—typically on the ovaries and fallopian tubes and

inside the pelvis—causing intense pain as it continues to grow and shed with nowhere to go. This condition is called endometriosis. (Read more about this in Chapter 4.)

FALLOPIAN TUBES AND OVARIES

The 4-inch-long fallopian tubes essentially collect an egg from the ovary next to it and deliver it to the uterus in a process called ovulation. Your ovaries are about an inch in size and have two jobs: The first is to release hormones like the all-important estrogen, and the second is to produce eggs. Estrogen is responsible for a range of functions, like breast development and regulating the menstrual cycle, and is a key player in the reproductive cycle. Think of it as the queen E that is in charge of all things related to being female. Estrogen is also known as the female sex hormone. (More on the hormonal hall of fame in Chapter 2).

ADDITIONAL ANATOMY THAT YOU SHOULD KNOW

The vagina is not an island. When we are talking about sex and sexuality, there are other body parts that come into play and have a strong connection to your vagina. Your brain is one of them. As we are sure you know, the brain controls all of your bodily functions, fields input from your senses, and allows you to think, plan, and dream—all of which have an impact on your vagina. The way it works is, the sensory experiences you get from your genitals are interpreted by your brain, and the brain then releases the neurotransmitter dopamine that activates the reward center of the brain. That feedback loop of pleasure, chemicals, and lighting up the reward center of the brain keeps people going back for more when it comes to sex and orgasm. We'll talk more about this later, but your brain plays a big role in sexual behavior, activity, and fantasy. It is also possible that a higher sex drive originates in the brain.

Another part of your anatomy (well, two parts of your anatomy) figures in sex and sexuality and is also linked to having a vagina—although not everyone who has one has the other—breasts. Yep, the girls can be sensitive players when it comes to sex, and stimulation of breasts and nipples can lead to arousal, which in turn leads to your vagina getting ready for sex. They are all connected. Because we are focusing on the vagina in Vagina U, we won't go into too much depth on breasts except to say that you should do self-exams to help screen for breast cancer, know your family history of breast cancer, and ask your gyno about when you should have mammograms.

SELF-EXAMINATION

When was the last time you took a peek at your vulva or vagina? Never? Once a long time ago? Time to take a look. Women don't often know what they look like "down there" because so much of our sexual and reproductive anatomy is hidden away. And that which is hidden often seems forbidden, off-limits, or even dangerous. (Don't get us started on the ridiculous myth of the vagina having teeth. We kid you not. You can look it up!) But unless you are a contortionist, the only way to get a good visual of your labia and become familiar with your anatomy is to use a hand mirror. Breaking out a mirror and

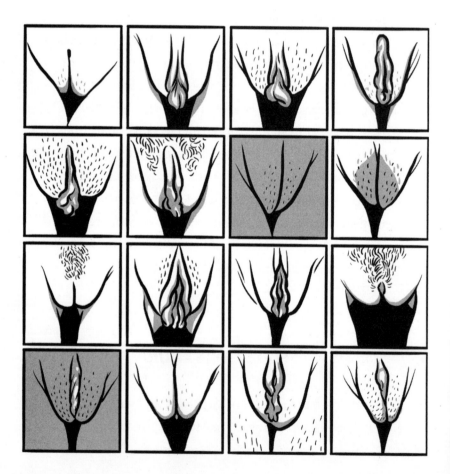

EX-QUEEF ME!

Your vagina can fart! Known as queefing, it is basically a trapped pocket of air being pushed out of your vagina and can happen during sex or during a workout. It's totally normal. If it is frequently happening to you during your workouts, a solution is to wear a tampon during your exercise routine, and that will block the air being expelled. If it happens during sex, well, it happens. Hopefully, you will both be so into what you are doing that your partner will not even notice. Or you will both be comfortable enough to laugh it off because—let's face it—it's a little funny!

---

taking a look is something you should do every once in a while.

Warning: Before you start searching for pictures on the Internet to see how your parts compare to other women, know that *everyone is different*. Repeat: *Everyone is different*. Unfortunately, porn has set a distorted standard for vaginal appearance that makes some women feel insecure about the appearance of their own vulvas. Rest assured, there is no "perfect" vulva or vagina. The color, size, and shape of a woman's labia is unique to her. You can have "big" lips or "small" lips. One side can be larger than the other side; one side can be smaller than the other side—in fact, most women do not have labia that are equal in size or perfectly symmetrical. If they are not equal and don't look like anyone else's, it is NBD. You are unique. Depending on your own skin tone, the color of your vulva and labia can vary from pink to dark brown and be any shade in between. Your genitals are like any other part of your anatomy in that they are generally the same as everyone else's but also unique to you.

For example, everyone's fingers have similar form and function, but their appearance, shape, size, and color are yours and yours alone.[1, 2, 3]

Just as the appearance, shape, and size of your vulva and labia are unique to you, so is the shape and size of your vagina. Many women worry that they are too big or too small, too wide or too narrow, but there actually isn't much difference among vaginal canals. "Tightness" or "looseness" is all relative. Your state of arousal, particular positions, and the anatomy of your partner (or shape of sex toys) can made a difference in how tight or loose you feel to yourself or your partner. Contrary to popular belief, frequent sex or sex with a partner with a large penis will not leave your vagina in a permanently stretched-out state. Your versatile vagina has the ability to expand to accommodate anything from a large penis to a baby! And despite what you may have heard, women who have given birth aren't too stretched out after delivering a baby to enjoy sex either. The vagina is pretty flexible and, yes, while it can expand to allow a baby to be born, it does not stay in that expanded state forever. As you heal after childbirth, the muscles and tissues often revert to the way they were before you pushed the baby into the world. In Chapter 5, we'll get into how and why there can be issues with your vagina, but for now, know that the muscles and tissues of the vagina are very adaptive and become lubricated and loose for vaginal penetration but at the same time remain tight to promote pleasure.

Unless you have pain or discomfort during penetrative sex or can't insert a tampon, you are in all likelihood completely within the realm of normal when it comes to the length, width, and "tightness" of your vagina.

WORK IT OUT

The vagina is a powerful muscle that, like any muscle in your body, can improve its function through exercise. You have probably already heard of Kegel exercises to strengthen the pelvic floor—that's the group of muscles that supports your uterus,

---

ANATOMICALLY CORRECT

In news that sounds more like science fiction, but is in reality science fact, a team of researchers from Northwestern University, the University of Illinois at Chicago, and Draper University has developed a three-dimensional working model of the female reproductive system including ovaries, fallopian tubes, a cervix, and a uterus made from human and mouse tissue. Not only is it anatomically correct, it can simulate a 28-day menstrual cycle and pregnancy hormones. Tissue can grow, and hormonal signaling operates the way it does in a woman's body. Known as Evatar—"Eve" combined with the word "avatar," meaning the digital representation of a person—the lab model can be used to test drugs and try to find solutions for health issues like endometriosis, infertility, and fibroids. It will also revolutionize the way that cancer is studied, allowing researchers to study the whole system as opposed to just the individual parts.[4]

bladder, small intestine, and rectum—to prevent leaking pee when you sneeze or losing your strong grip during sex. Exercising your vag with Kegels are a great way to tone the muscles of your pelvic floor, which is helpful for stopping the leaks but also for improving orgasm. Next time you go to the bathroom, you can figure out which muscles are doing the work by stopping your pee midstream (this is not something you should do all the time, as it's not good for your bladder, but it is okay just to figure out which muscles you need to be working). Once you have identified the muscles, then you can do Kegel exercises to get them in shape. For a few minutes each day, you can engage the muscles and hold them for 5 to 10 seconds, then release. These daily squeezes can lead to more intense orgasms. And who could say no to that?

If you want to take it to the next level, you can use vaginal barbells, Kegel exercise weights, or Kegel trainers. These are weights or devices that you insert into your vagina that require you to contract the muscles to keep the weight from sliding out. Some have apps to track your progress and some even vibrate! Over time, whether you use weights or not, you can increase your pelvic floor power and look forward to an increase in pleasure to go with it!

WHAT'S IN A NAME?

Recently there has been a movement to reclaim the use of the word *pussy* and move it away from being a derogatory term to one of power and protest. The euphemisms for female genitalia are endless, and while they are sometimes fun to throw around when chatting with girlfriends and being silly, it's important to be aware of the impact of failing to use the proper anatomical terminology when discussing women's bodies. Leah Millheiser, MD, ob-gyn and chief scientific officer for Nuelle, feels that it's important to normalize the word *vagina* because her concern is that by not saying it, we are making it a shameful taboo and communicating that message to young women and girls. In an interview, she said, "We can say *erectile dysfunction* very easily, we can say *penis* very easily, but we don't have that same opportunity to say *vagina*. So you're promoting shame in young women. We know from research that you actually reduce a young girl's willingness to report sexual abuse when she doesn't know proper genital terminology. So we really need to look at this from a public health perspective of what impact the incorrect terminology is having on young women."[5]

So let's lay off beaver, cooter, honeypot, box, and all of the other cringe-worthy and creative names that we've called it and start calling a vulva a vulva and a vagina a vagina, k?

VAGINAS AGE, TOO

When we talk about aging, we often speak of graying hair, aching backs, smile lines, and crow's-feet, but we don't often think of our genitals aging. Of course they do, however, right along with the rest of us.

IN YOUR TWENTIES

All of your internal reproductive organs have reached their full size and won't change significantly as time goes on once you reach your twenties. The only aspect of your anatomy that may change is your labia: The older you get, the less fat you have in your genitals, and both the labia majora and minora can become a little thinner, more fragile, and prone to injury.

IN YOUR THIRTIES

Your next decade of your thirties can have an impact on hormones. The fluctuation in your hormones at this age can actually lead to your labia minor becoming a little bit darker in color. Nothing dramatic, and you'd need your hand mirror or a particularly detail-oriented long-term partner to notice, but it happens. Good old hormones.

Also, by this age many women have given birth: The uterus has ballooned to watermelon proportions during pregnancy, and during vaginal delivery the vagina has been stretched to the point of tearing for many women. It returns to its original size within 6 weeks after birth.

IN YOUR FORTIES

When you reach your forties, although you still may be having a period, your egg supply (that's essentially been with you since you were born) will begin to diminish. Many women also make a stop at perimenopause as their fertility and menstrual cycles wind down.

As you age, those hormones that have been driving all things in the reproductive area, particularly estrogen, can decrease and can disrupt the pH balance in your vagina. The walls of the vagina can also thin and become dry, so use personal lubricant to keep things supple and—here's a tough assignment—have plenty of sex to keep your systems primed. Be sure to use water-based lube, as the thin, dry walls of the vagina can be damaged if they do not have enough moisture.

IN YOUR FIFTIES

Your period may fade away around age 50 or so, and you will be in full-blown menopause. You are officially in menopause when you have not had a period for 12 months. Because your reproductive organs are held in place by muscles and tendons, anything that can weaken those muscles can lead to discomfort or bladder leakage. Unfortunately, as you age you can lose muscle tone and elasticity of ligaments and tendons. Your defense against drooping reproductive organs is Kegels. Do them often and keep your pelvic floor strong and supportive.[6]

VAGINOPLASTY

You can get plastic surgery for just about any part of your anatomy, so it is no surprise that there are specialized surgical
procedures—vaginoplasty or vaginal rejuvenation for the
vagina, and labiaplasty for, you guessed it, the labia.

Women sometimes choose to have a procedure that will
reduce the size and change the appearance of their labia minora.
Reasons for having the surgery can include having labia that
protrude or are uneven, or because their size leads to rubbing,
chaffing, and discomfort. Some serious cyclists have had labia
reduction surgery to stop the discomfort they feel from spending so much time in the saddle.

Vaginoplasty or vaginal rejuvenation surgery is done to make
the vagina "tighter" and potentially lead to more pleasure
during sex. Women may seek this procedure after childbirth or
even as they age to correct what they may feel is a "loose"
vagina. You should know that the American College of Obstetricians and Gynecologists (ACOG) challenges the claim that the
surgery can restore sensitivity.[7]

Whether you are pro plasty or against it, it's important to
remember that everyone is different. You will need to discuss
your concerns with your gynecologist and then with a plastic
surgeon to determine if either of these surgeries is something
that would be appropriate for your situation. As with any surgery you undertake, you need to understand fully what the procedure is for, be confident in the expertise and experience of
your doctor or surgeon (your surgeon should be board certi-

fied), what the surgery will do, how much it will cost, what the recovery is like, and what you can expect in terms of healing and the ultimate results.

Another treatment that some women are using to improve their genitals and their ability to achieve orgasm is something called the O-Shot. The shot is basically platelet-rich plasma extracted from your own blood, then injected into your clitoris and vagina. Typically done for women in menopause or those who have trouble orgasming, the theory behind the shot is that it will give a boost to stem cell growth, allow tissue to grow, and get you more sensitive and able to orgasm.[8]

Your internal and external anatomy is impressively designed to serve a range of functions from pleasure to reproduction, and knowing where the parts are and how they work puts you in charge of your sexual and reproductive self. Knowing what your girl parts are called contributes to ownership and understanding your body as well as better control over your medical care and sexual health. While it can be playful and fun to have nicknames for your vulva or vagina, when it comes down to it, you should know the real deal.

Let's honor our bodies with knowing the right names. After all, if your name is Jane, and I always call you Ann, we could never have a very good relationship, could we? So if you retain nothing else from this chapter, remember: When you say "vulva" and I say "vagina," we are actually talking about two different part of a woman's anatomy.

2

YOUR PERIOD 101: WHY, WHEN, AND HOW TO DEAL

JUST LIKE THE VAGINA, periods are also a taboo subject. Who hasn't shamefully stuffed tampons into pockets and up sleeves on the way to the bathroom? Women work on the unobtrusive pad pass to needy friends. A woman will say she must have eaten something bad to cover for cramps and bloat. In short, women just don't talk about periods. Is it because periods = blood and blood = icky? Does everyone think that periods are gross even though they are a monthly part of life?

While most women can move through the world as usual while menstruating, from running corporations to running in marathons—just watch a tampon commercial and see all of those smiling women wearing white—there are still some women and girls today who are separated from their communities during that time of the month. According to a UNESCO report,

MODERN RED TENTS

According to an ancient Hindu practice of *Chhaupadi* (a word that translates to "untouchable being"), the touch of a menstruating woman can wilt crops and dry up wells. And although the practice is banned in Nepal, women and girls all over the country are confined to cowsheds or makeshift huts and fed only certain foods such as salted bread and rice during their period and after childbirth. Live in the city and don't have a shed? Well, just rent a separate apartment a few days per month. Not only do these practices reinforce the damaging belief that periods are something dirty to be ashamed of and prevent gender parity, but they put these women and girls in physical danger through poor sanitation and lack of access to medical care.[2]

1 in 10 girls in sub-Saharan Africa misses school during her period. This can add up to missing over 20 percent of the school year and sometimes causes girls to drop out altogether.[1]

One way to help those girls is to brush up on period facts so that the women in this generation and the next are empowered to view their period not as an obstacle or barrier but as a biological function and nothing be ashamed of at the least, and an empowering, creative force at the best!

BACK TO HEALTH CLASS

Raise your hand if you enjoy getting your period. Anyone with a hand in the air? Anyone? No? Not surprising. Periods can be messy, inconvenient, unpredictable, painful, and a monthly reminder of . . . that you'll get it again in another month? Who needs it? Well, once most people with a uterus hit puberty, periods are part of the package. And because having a menstrual cycle comes with the territory of being the proud owner of a vagina, it is good to understand just what is happening in your body month to month. It's also important to be familiar with your cycle if you want to get pregnant (or if you really don't) and in order to know what is normal for you so you can be alerted to any health concerns or issues.

Just in case you skipped health class, slept through health class, or never had health class to begin with (Catholic school, anyone?), here is a refresher on the typical menstrual cycle.

THE BASICS

Basically, the lining in the uterus builds up to be prepared to support a fertilized egg and nourish the growing fetus. If fertilization doesn't happen, the lining sheds and you have a period. Then the process starts all over again, and again, and again until you get pregnant (after which you start right up again) or age out completely when you hit menopause.

From your first period to your last, you can go through as many as 400 cycles. The days of a cycle are counted by starting with the first day of a period and ending the first day of the next one. While a typical cycle is 28 days, you may find that your cycle is anywhere from 21 to 35 days long—and the number of days in your cycle may vary from one month to the next (unless you are on a hormone-regulating form of birth control). It's good to know what your typical cycle is so that you can be aware of any significant changes. Plus, at every gynecologist appointment, your doctor will ask you the date of your last menstrual period, aka, the LMP. Many women like to keep track, one way or another, so that they are not taken by surprise and have to scramble for supplies. To keep you from counting on your fingers when the question comes up, there are a number of period tracker apps that you can download for free for use on your mobile phone, or you can do it the old-fashioned way and mark it on your calendar. It is no fun walking around with toilet tissue wadded up in your underwear because you lost track of when "Aunt Flo" is coming to visit. Should you be trying to become pregnant, keeping track of your period can help in

---

OVULATION CALCULATION

To find out which days of the month you are the most fertile, first track your period for a few months to get an average, each time recording the first day of your period as "day 1." Once you have that, delete 18 days from your shortest cycle and delete 11 days from your longest cycle. The days in between are the days you are most likely to get pregnant.[3] Because most women have a 28-day menstrual cycle, there are usually 6 days each month when you can get pregnant—the day you ovulate and the 5 days before. While not a reliable birth control method, this method can help you when you are looking to get in the family way!

achieving that goal because you'll know the days you are most fertile and need to get busy to make that baby!

Most periods last 3 to 5 days, and your flow can be light, heavy, or somewhere in between. Pretty simple, right? It's actually a little more complicated than that. What seems like a relatively basic operation is guided by some complex and finely tuned biological processes.

Here's what is going on behind the scenes:

Hormones are the key players in all things related to your period. Estrogen is prevalent in the first half of the cycle, progesterone is at its highest during the second half of your cycle, and testosterone is relatively constant throughout.

Estrogen, released by the ovary, signals the uterus to build up a lining (cells, tissue, and lots of blood vessels) in anticipation of a fertilized egg. While that is happening, the ovaries are triggered to release an egg (typically around day 14 of a 28-day cycle). The egg travels from the ovary to its nearest fallopian tube and on toward the uterus. If the egg encounters sperm and is fertilized, it will imbed itself in the lining of the uterus and begin developing into a baby. If fertilization does not take place, then the egg will not burrow into the uterine lining, the lining will begin to shed, and tissue and blood will flow out of the cervix into the vagina as your period.

Following are the highlights of an average cycle. Note that your cycle may be longer or shorter and not follow this cycle to the letter, even month to month. When it comes to all things period and all things hormonal, your normal is what you want to pay attention to and understand.

Day 1: First day of period.

Days 1–5: Bleeding.

Day 7. Bleeding will usually have stopped; hormone levels rise.

Days 7–14: Follicle in ovary develops (aka follicular stage).

Day 14: Follicle releases the egg and ovulation occurs; the egg travels to the uterus (aka luteal stage).

Days 18–23: Preperiod symptoms (including bloating, breakouts, and bad mood) set in; PMS.

Day 25: If the egg isn't fertilized, hormone levels drop and a period soon follows.

Day 28: Last day of cycle; next day will be your period.

Although the menstrual cycle seems relatively uncomplicated, things don't always follow the set pattern. You can be late, on time, miss a period; have superheavy flow, have virtually no flow; feel awful, feel fine; be on an emotional roller coaster or barely notice when you have your period. Your overall health and your environment can be factors that influence these changes, but at the end of the day, the timing, emotional and physical reactions, duration, and flow are largely dependent on how your body reacts to hormones.[4]

HORMONES

Coordinating complex processes like growth, metabolism, and fertility, hormones are the body's chemical messaging system.

They can influence the function of the immune system and even alter behavior. They were at work before you were born, coursing through your body and aiding in the development of your brain and reproductive system, making sure your arms grow to the same length, turning food into fuel, and getting ready to spring puberty on you when you least expect it.

Hormones allow the body to communicate, acting in response to signals from the brain and are secreted directly into the blood by the glands that produce and store them. These glands make up what is known as the endocrine system (*endocrine* means "secreting internally").[5]

Your cycle is controlled by the ebb and flow of hormones that are released in a pattern that repeats, in sequence, over the course of an average of 28 days. Because the 28-day cycle is roughly equivalent to the cycle of the moon, there is an erroneous belief that women's cycles are linked in some way to the lunar cycle. But before you start running naked in the forest worshipping lunar goddesses, remember that it's really your hormones and your brain that are in charge. Here is the list of the major players responsible for triggering changes in this particular part of your body.[6]

ESTROGEN

Estradiol—the most potent form of estrogen—prepares the uterus for conception. From your breasts to your bones, estrogen sends signals to every cell in your body to grow. When you maintain stable levels of this hormone, it can boost sex drive and immunity. When your levels are out of whack—such as when you are underweight and production halts, or when you are carrying too much weight and those extra fat cells cause your body to produce a type of estrogen that messes with estradiol—there are some pretty drastic results. High levels of estradiol can lead to severe PMS, fertility difficulties, and even breast cancer, while levels that are too low can lead to osteoporosis. Maintaining a healthy weight can help in supporting that balance.

PROGESTERONE

Each month, this hormone creates a cushy uterine lining (i.e., an embryo crib), and it triggers your period when no egg is implanted. Progesterone is responsible for the sounder sleep that many women experience right before their period as a result of its mild sedative effect, but it's also to blame for water retention, gassiness, and constipation around that same time . . . ugh. Many women who are trying to get pregnant turn to over-the-counter creams because of the belief that this hormone is so essential to achieving that goal. But studies show those creams are useless, while meditation for as little as 5 minutes per day could have some benefits when it comes to fertility.[7]

TESTOSTERONE

Testosterone is not just for guys! The androgen hormone supports regular ovulation and a hearty libido—yes, please! Levels that are too high can cause polycystic ovary syndrome—or PCOS—resulting in acne, dandruff, or dark hair in abnormal places (more about PCOS on page 38). Your overall sense of well-being and motivation can be obscured by low levels of this hormone, and increasing your intake of zinc-rich foods like hummus can increase levels. Striving for that beneficial body mass index is important here also, as testosterone in high levels is linked to obesity. And don't worry—you won't grow a beard, you'll just have more energy!

PROLACTIN

Made in the brain, prolactin controls egg release and stimulates breast-milk production in new moms. After childbirth, normal levels can help you ditch that baby weight! Sky-high levels of this hormone can stop your sex drive in its tracks and bring on menopause-like symptoms—a condition that, thankfully, is rare. Ovulation is suppressed by slightly elevated levels as well. Stress hormones such as cortisol and prolactin can spike as a result of less-than-ideal amounts of sleep. Commit to 7 to 8 hours of uninterrupted Z-catching every night to aid in achieving optimal hormone balance.

GNRH

Gonadotropin-releasing hormone (GnRH) is the link between the brain and the ovaries and assists in getting all systems go.

Much of the orchestration of the release of hormones occurs in the brain, where the pituitary gland is triggered to release the hormones that gets the ovaries to release the egg that is then open to being fertilized—or not, as the case may be.[8]

FSH/LH

Follicle-stimulating hormone (FSH) readies eggs for their big moment of fertilization, while luteinizing hormone (LH) releases them down the fallopian tubes and into the uterus. While a spike in FSH has been linked to memory problems, insomnia, and acne, balanced FSH/LH amounts can contribute to favorable progesterone levels. Alcohol can throw these two out of whack, so keep it at fewer than two drinks per day.

MITTLESCHMERZ

Some women get a little pain, almost like a pinch in their side, when they ovulate. This is called *mittleschmerz*, from the German word for "middle pain." It's not too extreme and usually doesn't require treatment. A heating pad and/or aspirin, ibuprofen, or acetaminophen will likely ease any discomfort if you feel treatment is necessary.

Who hasn't blamed hormones for something? Feeling crabby, bloated, or out of sorts is common in the hormone blame game—especially when it comes to PMS. But look at it this way: Hormones are an incredibly powerful and well-orchestrated force that keeps you "all systems go" and your body in balance. Unfortunately, anything that has such a fine-tuned operation can be thrown off kilter by behavior and lifestyle. Being under- or overweight, poor sleep, bad nutrition, or engaging in too much exercise can disrupt your hormones function. The good news is that you don't have to be at the mercy of hormones gone wild. There is much you can do to get your hormones back in balance and well regulated. Happy hormones = happy you!

WHEN YOU GET YOUR PERIOD

Most women have a story about that first time. For some it was embarrassing and confusing—like your mom made your dad congratulate you or you bled through your shorts in gym class—and for others their first thought was: "Well, it's about time!" Whether long anticipated or something no one thought to mention, a first period often comes as a surprise, although there are preliminary warnings that it is on its way. Breasts as well as armpit and pubic hair usually make their appearance before the menarche—the formal name for your first period. The average age for a first period in the United States is 12 to 14 years, but you may have started earlier or later. In the United States, puberty—and as a result, periods—have been trending earlier, and there are girls as young as 10 who begin menstruating. Obesity may lead to early—or "precocious"—

NOT A GIRL, NOT YET A WOMAN

While determining the causes and medical repercussions of early puberty in girls is important work for scientists, what may be even more important is how we treat these vulnerable children who may be easily mistaken for women based on their appearance. The teasing and innuendos are bad enough, and the unwanted attention can be confusing and emotionally upsetting for these girls, who are simply victims of their own biology. Earlier sex ed in schools as well as more open, honest conversations about biology, sexuality, respect, and bullying could go a long way toward protecting them.[10]

puberty as a result of excess fat producing heightened levels of estrogen in the child's body that signals early development. But as more studies are done on this issue, researchers are finding that increased levels of stress in families as well as exposure to certain chemicals in the environment or in food may also be to blame.[9] The only thing that we know for certain about this issue is that we don't really know anything for certain, unfortunately.

REGULARITY

As we've mentioned, the average cycle for a period is 28 days, but unless you are on hormone-based birth control, the number of days in your cycle can be longer or shorter than this and, just to keep things interesting, you may not have the same number of days in your cycle each month. The length of your period can vary based on a number of factors, but age is one of the biggest ones. A teenager may have a shorter, longer, or erratic cycle than a 20- or 30-year-old. Cycle length can shorten and become more predictable as you get older, but numerous influences on regularity can cause your periods to be late, irregular, or ghost you and not show up at all.

LATE, MISSING, AND IRREGULAR PERIODS

If your period is late, your first thought may be, "Am I pregnant?" If you are sexually active and even if you have been using birth control, pregnancy is a possibility. However, before you rush out and take a pregnancy test or frantically call Planned Parenthood, it can be worth sitting tight for a bit to see if your period is simply a little slow in coming. Sometimes periods arrive fashionably late! If you are confident that you could not possibly be pregnant, know that there are other scenarios that can cause your period to go AWOL. In a number of cases, not getting a period is nature's way of making sure you don't get pregnant, because being in a stressful environment or having compromised health is not an ideal situation for becoming pregnant and having a baby. In addition to missed periods in these cases, your period can be irregular or you can experience spotting/breakthrough bleeding or have lighter or heavier periods than normal.

If you're awaiting a stubbornly late period, ask yourself these questions to see if you can narrow down the culprit before you start stockpiling diapers or rushing to your doctor's office in a panic.

- Have you been under a lot of stress lately?
  Being under stress can cause a skipped period or mess with its arrival time. If you are dealing with a challenging or life-changing event (a death in the family, moving, marriage, or new job), the stress may be the cause of a missed period.
- Have you been exercising more than usual?
  Training intensely for an event can interrupt your cycle. Marathon training can make menstruation run off: Due to the strain that excessive exercise puts on the body, your body may think you are living in a stressful environment. When the body is under stress, it assumes that the environment you are in is not a friendly place for a child and makes it less likely that you will conceive.
- Have you recently lost a lot of weight?
  If you have a low body mass index (BMI under 19), you will likely not get your period. Estrogen, the hormone that drives all things period-related, is stored in fat. If you do not have enough fat, you will not have enough estrogen in your body, and you will not get your period. Women who are anorexic typically stop menstruating.
- Are you overweight?
  If you are overweight, extra fatty tissue on your body can bring more estrogen into your system that can mess with

your cycle. Diet, exercise, and birth control may help to regulate and stabilize your period.

- Have you recently stopped taking birth control or have you started a new method of birth control?

  Some forms of birth control can cause your period to stop completely. Sometimes when you stop using a form of birth control, it can take some time for your periods to resume. Additionally, a new form of birth control can lead to breakthrough bleeding or spotting. Getting a period will usually resolve once you have been using the birth control through a couple of cycles, but if it does not, speak to your health-care provider.

- Could it be your thyroid?

  If you have any type of thyroid issue—hypothyroidism or hyperthyroidism—these diseases can mess with your cycle. If you are being treated for a thyroid condition, talk to your doctor about your missed periods or any changes you experience with your period.

- Could it be PCOS?

  Caused by a hormone imbalance (a surplus of testosterone), polycystic ovary syndrome can make you miss your period or can cause irregular periods. Symptoms of PCOS (in addition to not having periods) include hair growth, acne, and weight gain. Medication, weight loss, and going on birth control can help regulate the hormonal imbalance causing PCOS.[11]

- Is it the female athlete triad?

  This triple whammy is usually brought on by disordered

PCOS—POLYCYSTIC OVARY SYNDROME

Between 5 to 10 percent of women of childbearing age in the United States, or roughly 5 million, have PCOS, but because many of these women are typically irregular or miss periods, their doctors might not connect the hallmark symptoms or chalk it up to stress, leaving more than 50 percent of sufferers misdiagnosed. PCOS is one of the most misunderstood disorders impacting modern women.

Along with the irregular or missed periods because of nonovulation that characterize PCOS, women with PCOS often experience weight gain, hair growth on the face or other parts of the body in a male hair-growth pattern, extreme pelvic pain, very heavy periods, fatigue, excessive acne, and sleep issues. Some, but not all, women will develop the ovarian cysts for which the disorder is named. PCOS is the leading cause of female infertility in developed countries, so if you have many of these symptoms you should consult with your doctor.

To get diagnosed, you will have your blood tested to determine your hormone levels. Usually PCOS causes abnormally high testosterone levels. You may also receive an ultrasound to assess whether or not you have cysts built up on your ovaries. These cysts can burst and be extremely painful.

Although there is no cure, birth control pills can help get the ovaries back on schedule, regulate periods, and suppress elevated levels of testosterone, which is what can be causing unwanted hair growth. Weight loss can also work to reduce symptoms. Although PCOS can lead to difficulty conceiving, fertility treatments can be used in order to get pregnant.[12]

eating, including excessive dieting (or excessive exercise), loss of periods (amenorrhea), and loss of bone density. If you are a female athlete and stop getting your period, talk to your doctor, as you may be at risk for fractures or broken bones as well.[13]

- Could it be perimenopause?

The beginnings of perimenopause can cause all sorts of havoc with your period—light bleeding, heavy bleeding, or no bleeding. If you are having period problems, are over 40, and also experience night sweats, hot flashes, or mood swings, speak with your doctor about the possibility of perimenopause. Note that the average age for perimenopause is 40, but it can happen as early as 30.

- Could it be abnormal growths?

Your period can get a little wacko if you have any abnormal growths in your uterus or ovaries. These growths can be anything from cysts to polyps to fibroids. Again, anything that seems out of the ordinary for your cycle should be brought to the attention of your gyno.

- Do you have a chronic disease?

If your body is stressed due to a chronic disease or disorder, you may skip periods or miss periods altogether. Speak with your doctor if irregular periods could be a side effect of your disease/disorder or medications you may be taking to treat your issue.

- Could you have an STI/STD?

Bacterial and viral infections can cause spotting (along with discharge and discomfort), so if you are spotting frequently, work with your doctor to determine if a sexually transmitted infection/sexually transmitted disease (STI/STD) is the cause and get the correct antibiotic or antiviral treatment—your partner, too!

The main thing to remember is that while missing a period or having irregular periods can be completely normal, it can also be a sign of a range of health issues and is definitely worth mentioning to your doctor. Keep in mind that cycles do not always run like clockwork, but you know best how often your period shows up and how long it stays, so if it varies from *your* norm it's worth having it checked out, especially if it veers off of the norm for a couple of months. And by checked out, we don't mean a late-night panic session with Dr. Google; instead, make an appointment with your gynecologist or other health-care provider—in person, in the office, with you in the paper gown and a real live doctor answering your questions and giving you care.

PERIOD SIDE EFFECTS

Hormonal changes in your body aren't responsible only for regulating your menstrual cycle—they can have an impact on other parts of your body as well. An uptick in progesterone can lead to hair being oily while also adding some extra shine to your skin (and hello, breakouts!). You can have bloating and water retention that make the waistband of your jeans feel smaller and the number on the scale grow larger. Hormonal fluctuations can cause cravings for all things salty, greasy, or chocolate (pick your pleasure/poison!), which contributes to weight gain as well. And don't forget about how tender your breasts can get—thanks, hormones! You can become more emotional and find yourself crying at things that wouldn't ordinarily release the waterworks—like that really cute video of otters holding hands as they sleep. The hormonal changes that occur during your menstrual cycle are inevitable, but if you maintain your exercise routine, get sleep, and eat healthfully, you can reduce the impact of the side effects and have a slightly more pleasant pre-period and period experience.

PERIOD PROBLEMS—AND SOLUTIONS!

It's not enough to cope with bloodflow every month, but many women also experience a range of symptoms before or during their periods that are inconvenient at the least and painful at the most. No matter what the severity of your symptoms, there are multiple strategies for dealing with them ranging from all natural (including herbs or movement) to medications (over-the-counter or prescription) that you may find helpful. Following are some common, specific symptoms and some troubleshooting techniques that you can try when you are hit with them.

Bloating ·
Bloating is also caused by . . . wait for it . . . hormone changes. Surprised? Bloating is really a result of the same fluid retention

---

IN SYNC

The next time you are tempted to think, "Are our cycles synced up?" when your BFF asks to borrow a tampon and you have one because you have your period, too, think again! What's probably happening is that your cycles are overlapping so you have your periods at the same time on a particular day this month, but not that your hormonal and ovulation cycles are identical. Or, if you are on the Pill, you may be starting your packs on the same day (many women start on Sunday) and thus will be going through your pill-driven cycle at the same time.[14, 15]

---

that gets your boobs feeling achy. Belly bloating can cause discomfort, your favorite pair of jeans may feel tighter, and the number on your scale may rise. It's all temporary but not much fun. Strategies for beating the bloat include eating a balanced diet that does not include a lot of salt, increasing your water consumption, reducing caffeine, reducing alcohol, taking an over-the-counter diuretic, and engaging in exercise. If your fluid retention is extreme, speak to your doctor, as there may be prescription meds that will help with the issue.

Breakouts

And you thought that once high school was over, pimples would be a thing of the past. Well, blemishes usually pop up in the week preceding your period because those hormones are at it again and making your skin a bit oilier. Although the cause of the pimples is internal hormonal changes, you can take steps to address your exterior. The trick to dealing with these period pimples is to be proactive and step up your face-cleansing routine. Use a slightly stronger cleanser, use a lighter moisturizer, try a lighter hand with foundation, or try a facial peel or mask. You know your skin. If you have delicate skin, treat it gently. Your mom was right: no pimple popping! If breakouts become a major issue, then you can work with your dermatologist to keep your skin healthy and glowing all month long. You can also consult with your doctor about your birth control method and if it may be a contributor to your breakouts.

Cramps

While they may seem to add insult to injury each month, cramps are actually a signal that your uterus is contracting to shed the lining that comes out as menstrual blood. But just because your body is doing what it is supposed to do doesn't make it any easier on you. Besides taking an over-the-counter painkiller, you can try heat on your abdomen, as that will help dilate blood vessels and get things moving. Some women swear by moist heat and say nothing helps more than a hot-water bottle or even a warm bath. While it may be tempting to lie on the couch with a heating pad clutched to your abdomen and binge-watch Netflix, getting off the couch and moving can actually help make the cramps go away. Exercise not only keeps you healthy in general but it promotes optimum bloodflow, and if you exercise enough so that your endorphins kick in, then your cramps will soon be forgotten. If an over-the-counter medicine

(continued on page 46)

YOGA MOVES FOR COPING WITH CRAMPS

Yoga exercises are great for relaxation and for lengthening and strengthening muscles. When it comes to coping with cramps, there are a number of yoga moves that can bring relief. If you've never done yoga before, take a class at your local yoga studio, health club, or gym. You can also find yoga instructional videos online.

These three exercises can be done on a mat, or you can lay a towel on the floor (just be sure it won't slip) or do them on a deep carpet or rug. Wear loose, comfortable clothing and be barefoot.

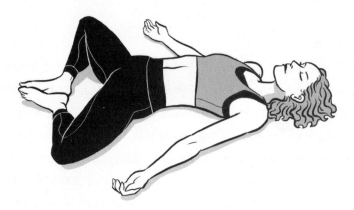

Reclining Goddess

Sit on the floor with the soles of your feet together and your legs in a diamond shape. Let your knees fall out to the sides and lie back, spreading your arms out to the sides, palms up. Feel free to place yoga blocks or pillows under your knees if you feel pulling in the groin or hips, as well as under your back or neck if you experience discomfort Hold this hip-opening position for 1 minute.

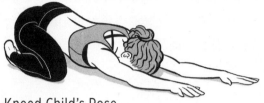

Wide-Kneed Child's Pose

Kneel on your mat with your knees a little wider than hip-distance apart. Fold at the waist and release forward, extending your arms in front of you until they reach the mat while at the same time lowering your butt toward your feet (it's okay if your butt and feet aren't in direct contact). The palms of your hands and your forehead will be touching the mat or floor in front of you. Settle your hips into a comfortable position, enjoying the gentle, restorative stretch, and hold for at least 1 minute.

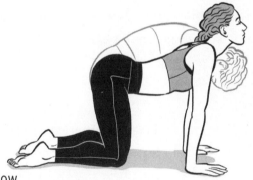

Cat/Cow

This move gives you a midsection massage that can flex and stretch muscles and vanquish cramps. Get on your hands and knees on your mat with hands about shoulder-width apart and knees about hip-distance apart. Inhale as you tuck your tailbone under, rounding your upper back, drawing your belly in, and dropping your head for cat pose, then exhale as you lift your head and tailbone so your belly lowers toward the floor for cow pose. Cycle through these poses slowly, feeling the stretch and focusing on your breath, 10 times.[16]

doesn't help with the pain, it is worth a call to your doctor to rule out any other health issues that could be causing your severe discomfort (see pages 44–45 for yoga moves to help with cramps).

Emotional Upheaval

You may know your period is coming when the image of the little kitten who needs a home on that late-night commercial causes you to break down in tears right there on your couch. We don't want to promote stereotypes, but many women have their emotions thrown into overdrive because of the hormonal fluctuations of the menstrual cycle. A solution may lie in what you are eating. Your emotions can be influenced by high or low blood sugar, so deny those cravings for junk food and dig into complex carbs (whole grains and vegetables) so you can level out your blood sugar *and* your emotions.

Food Cravings

Food cravings are very common prior to periods, and they are usually for food items that are not good for you. Ever heard of anyone having a preperiod craving for a salad? We haven't either. The sad fact is that some common cravings can contribute to your discomfort, both physical and, as we mentioned previously, emotional. Neurotransmitters and your old pal hormones are working to make you want to inhale that bag of chips. Resist! Some people crave salty and some people crave sweet. Some crave both. For some women, a strong craving for chocolate is a clue that their period is on its way. Cravings are tough to resist, but they can be tamed so that they don't overwhelm you and trigger other symptoms. The key is to give in to the craving occasionally and have a bit of what you are longing for and savor it. One piece of quality chocolate (especially dark chocolate) that you allow to melt in your mouth may conquer the craving, and you won't find yourself facedown in a pan of brownies later. The big bag of chips that is calling your name can be cut down to size—quite literally—if you take a baggie or small bowl and give yourself a serving (it can be generous, don't worry) and then put the big bag back on the pantry shelf. If you start on the big bag, you will find yourself at the bottom of it in no time, and you won't be doing yourself any favors when it comes to other symptoms, as salt can spark bloating and breast tenderness.

Headache

Headaches are triggered by a shift in the hormones estrogen and progesterone. Some women will get a headache a few days before their period when the estrogen in their body drops. It's annoying, but you can treat it like any other headache with whatever typically works for you, including ibuprofen, acetaminophen, or naproxen, and it should go away. Sometimes a cool compress on your forehead will make you feel better. You can also get gel headache masks at the drugstore or online that you put in the refrigerator or freezer and place over your eyes for cooling and soothing. Another strategy is to try a warm compress on your forehead (some of the gel headache masks can be heated) or use a heating pad on your neck. Some women find that having some caffeine can bring relief, but be careful: Too much caffeine can also set off headaches.

In other women, menstruation can be a trigger for migraines.

Migraines are the mother of all headaches and are so severe that they can prevent you from following your usual daily activities. Migraines are usually throbbing, on one side of the head, and can come with nausea, light sensitivity, or sensitivity to sound. Menstrual migraine can happen if you are already a migraine sufferer, or you may get these horrible headaches only when you have your period. Occasionally your doctor may recommend a type of oral birth control with a small amount of hormone during the placebo days of the period that can alleviate menstrual migraine. If you already get migraines, then you can treat the migraine with your usual medication as prescribed by your doctor. You can also try self-help strategies like lying quietly in a darkened room, using hot or cold compresses (whichever feels better to you), or drinking a little bit of caffeine. If you consistently get severe, debilitating headaches right before or with your period, you should keep track of when they occur and how they coincide with your period so you can talk to your doctor and see if you need a prescription medication for coping with the headaches. Your doctor may also review your birth control method, as the hormones contained in them may be triggering headaches. We'll cover more on birth control and the impacts they have on your body and mood in Chapter 3.

Other methods of managing headaches include acupressure. You can purchase acupressure bands over the counter that are usually sold for preventing seasickness, but a headache with nausea feels pretty much the same on land or on sea, and these bands can definitely help. Relaxation exercises or biofeedback has also given women relief from headaches.[17]

RELAXATION TECHNIQUES

It's normal to respond to pain by tensing up, but the problem is that tensing up can make the pain worse. To alleviate the pain of headache, you can practice some simple relaxation techniques. The first is working with your breathing. Taking deep, slow breaths as you allow your abdomen to expand and then exhaling slowly can bring calm and relaxation. You can take in a deep breath to the count of five and let it out slowly to the count of five. Breathing in through the nose and out through the mouth can regulate your breath. Another headache helper is engaging in movement to relieve muscle tension. Have you found that your neck and shoulders get stiff and tight when you have a headache? Simply rotate your head from side to side and free up the neck muscles (don't push or stretch so far that you cause further pain). Additionally, you can raise and lower your shoulders, squeezing your shoulders toward your ears and releasing them. Rolling your shoulders forward and back can also take some of the tension and tightness out of your muscles.

Heavy Flow

The amount of your flow can fluctuate from period to period, and your level of flow may be different from a friend's period. To assess if there is a problem, ask yourself if the flow is heavier than normal for you. If you are going through period supplies much faster than normal or if the flow is so heavy that you need to stay home from work, you should contact your doctor. A potential measure for heavy flow would be needing to change your tampon or pad every hour for several hours a day or for multiple days. Your doctor can evaluate you for any potential health issues. Going on birth control can help keep the flow in check.

Also, if you have a heavier flow, you may see dark clots of blood when you change your pad or tampon. If they are smaller than the size of a grape, it is fine and is just due to the blood flowing from your vagina so quickly that it doesn't have time to coagulate. Blood clots bigger than a plum should be discussed with your doctor. You may need a medication to help with the issue, and you may need to be treated for anemia because of the excessive blood loss you are experiencing monthly due to heavy flow.

Muscle Ache

A common symptom many women experience during their periods is muscle ache, most often in their backs. An over-the-counter anti-inflammatory medication can help, as can a heating pad, hot-water bottle, stretching, or gentle massage.

Odor

You may notice a different odor down there when you are on your period. It's usually a result of a combination of bacteria, sweat, and blood. The best defense for offensive odor is to change your pad or tampon regularly and clean your vulva with gentle soap and water frequently. Although you may be tempted to reach for douches, they can be irritating and cause more problems for this sensitive area. In fact, the vagina itself—the interior part of your lady bits—is a bit like a self-cleaning oven, and adding even just soap and water up inside can damage the delicate balance. So don't douche! (See Chapter 5 for more on these topics.)

Poop Problems

At the onset of your period, your body releases prostaglandins, which cause smooth muscle (like the uterus) to contract, and guess what is also made of smooth muscle? Yes, your digestive tract. So you may pass gas more frequently than usual, poop more, or have loose poop during your period.[18] And just because bodies are interesting, you can also be constipated. Your diet during your period, as it does at other times in your life, can influence your bowel movements. So try to keep healthy foods on your plate and, as tempting as they are, skip the deep-fried and supersweet items. Drinking lots of water and increasing your fiber intake can help. Taking an ibuprofen 24 hours before your period starts may resolve bowel issues.[19]

Sore Boobs

Some women experience sore breasts that are caused by the hormonal shifts of the menstrual cycle that in turn trigger fluid retention. You can try wearing a different bra, taking over-the-counter anti-inflammatory medications, and cutting back on caffeine. Sometimes standing in a warm shower can bring relief. If you are on birth control, the hormones may be affecting your breasts, so it's worth bringing up the soreness with your gynecologist. If you engage in high-impact sports, be sure to wear a very supportive sports bra, because tender breasts + jumping up and down or running can = further discomfort. If you typically experience tender breasts before or at the onset of your period, take note if you feel a different level of pain at another stage in your cycle, find a lump, or have nipple discharge—these changes warrant talking with your doctor.

Weight Gain

Joy of joys, having your period can help you pack on 5 or more pounds! Fun! Bloat and water retention (thanks, hormones) are the biggest culprit, but the cravings for fried foods, salty foods, and chocolate can inspire you to indulge and add to the belly bulge.

HERBS FOR WHAT AILS YOU

There are a number of herbs you can take during your period to help alleviate symptoms of headache, bloating, irritability, and more.[20] Some herbs many women use and the symptoms they relieve are:

Chasteberry: Bloating, breast pain
Dong quai: Insomnia, cramps, and headache
Lemon balm: Anxiety
St. John's wort: Depression
Ginkgo biloba: Mood changes and water retention

Remember that herbs can interact with medications, so be sure to tell your health-care provider if you are taking any herbal treatments. A word of caution: St. John's wort can make some birth control pills less effective, so share the information about what you are taking so you and your health-care professional take the proper steps to keep you on a healthy path.[21]

PMS-PREMENSTRUAL SYNDROME

If we could ban anyone from asking "Are you on your period?" whenever a woman is grumpy, cranky, or otherwise out of sorts, we would. Especially when it's another women who asks the question. (What ever happened to the solidarity of sisterhood!?) Let's see if we can starve that stereotype and make it disappear. Honestly, though, the stereotype exists because so many women feel crabby before getting their periods—typically they are fatigued, bloated, or irritable. Throw into the mix sore boobs, headaches, cramps, weight gain, and breakouts, and you have a recipe for some serious grumps. And those are just a few of the physical joys of impending periods—the emotional ones include irritability, depression, brain fog, and more.

The dreaded symptoms of PMS typically rear their ugly heads at the end of your cycle, just before menstruation starts. Have you ever caught yourself wondering why you were feeling crummy, biting the head off of your partner, or craving chocolate and then realized that time of the month is just about now? Well, that could be PMS.

While many women have some or all of these symptoms, and can usually shake them off, if these physical and psychological experiences are kicked up a notch, they are an indication of PMS. PMS, in case you didn't know, stands for premenstrual syndrome and is a collection of symptoms that show up a week or so before your period and can be severe enough to interfere in your normal day-to-day functioning with work, friends, or family. As in mood swings so severe that you can't cope in any form of relationship at work or at home. PMS is a giant step beyond just being "hormonal."

Many women will say they have PMS, although to truly have it, you need to be diagnosed by a doctor, and that involves you telling her about the regularity and duration of your symptoms, providing a health history, and answering some lifestyle questions—stress? smoking? diet? family history?—as well as undergoing a physical exam.

If you are diagnosed with PMS, some strategies can help. Actions you can take include quitting smoking, cutting back on caffeine, maintaining exercise, eating well, and getting enough sleep. In cases of more severe PMS, your doctor may prescribe birth control pills to level off hormonal fluctuations affecting your body, and she may suggest diuretics to deal with bloating or antidepressants to manage emotional symptoms.[22] Another approach gaining traction is to use medical marijuana to counter the symptoms of PMS. Medical marijuana has been prescribed for pain relief as well as to help stabilize mood (two of the major components of PMS). Heck, even Whoopi Goldberg has gotten in on the action and launched a company that sells products for combating PMS that contain medical marijuana; check out the Web site Whoopi & Maya (http://whoopiand-maya.com).

PMDD—PREMENSTRUAL DYSPHORIC DISORDER

For some women—3 to 9 percent of the population—the time before their periods goes well beyond PMS into premenstrual dysphoric disorder. The symptoms are similar to those of regular PMS, but they are in the extreme. PMDD kicks in after ovulation and lasts until a couple of days before you get your period. Depression, moodiness, and anxiety can be so severe as to impact daily life. The emotional changes are different from general depression or anxiety because they will come on at midcycle and go away once the period starts. If you experience emotional extremes during your cycle, the best way to pin down the where and when is to keep track in a journal, notebook, or smartphone what symptoms you experience, when they arrive, and how long they last. You can work with your doctor to strategize the best approach to treating the condition. Birth control pills can stabilize hormonal fluctuations, and your doctor may suggest the addition of an antidepressant to stabilize your mood. Exercise, relaxation techniques, and behavioral therapies can also help you deal.[23]

MENSTRUAL BLOOD

While some people may find themselves squeamish around blood, a lifetime of periods makes most women capable of telling the difference between blood from between their legs and blood that seeps from a wound. Each cycle, women lose from 4 tablespoons to as much as a cup of blood![24]

Menstrual blood is different from the blood in the rest of your body in that it doesn't clot easily so that it can flow out of your vagina—it will look different from the blood that comes from a cut, for example—and the way it looks can tell you a lot about your health. In fact, the American College of Obstetricians and Gynecologists recommends that the menstrual cycle be viewed as a vital sign the same way your blood pressure, pulse, and temperature are. Why? Because in addition to telling you whether you're pregnant or not, your period can provide essential insights into your hormone health—and as we know, hormones keep everything from your brain to your reproductive system running smoothly.[25]

You can learn a lot about your health and the health of your period from just the color of your menstrual blood alone! Here are some of the indicators of health that can show up in the color of your menstrual blood.

Bright Red

A hearty cranberry red color indicates a healthy flow for most women! Everyone's "normal" is a little different, but seeing this bright shade usually indicates that everything is going swimmingly. The consistency of your period blood shouldn't be watery but also shouldn't be quite as thick as ketchup.

Dark Brown

If yours appears to be dark brown (usually at the beginning of your period), not to worry, as this color is totally normal and a result of slow bloodflow. You may also notice clots when you are having a period that collect in your pad or tampon or drop into the toilet in the bathroom when you go. While they can freak you out a little, they typically occur because you are shedding your uterine lining quickly, and they usually accompany a heavy flow. If you consistently experience heavy flow and lots of clotting, have a conversation with your doctor to find the appropriate treatment.

Light Pink

Light pink may indicate that your estrogen levels are low, which can be caused by an increase in exercise, poor nutrition, PCOS, or perimenopause. Although it might feel like a break to skip your period while you are training for a marathon or just hitting the gym extra hard, low estrogen levels can increase your risk of osteoporosis if left untreated, so chat with your doctor if this seems like it's becoming an issue for you.

Pale and Watery

Anemia can make your periods very pale and watery. This can also be an indication of other nutritional deficiencies. On the other hand—somewhat confusingly—an iron deficiency can lead to superheavy flow that will soak through a pad or tampon in less than an hour, the need to change tampons or pads in the middle of the night, and feeling tired and unfocused, so speak with your doctor about having your iron levels checked in that case.

Jam-Colored with Clots

A sign that you have uterine fibroids or that your progesterone and estrogen balance is off (low progesterone and high estrogen) is period blood the color of jam with frequent clots. Note that some clotting is normal, but clots that are bigger than the size of a plum may be telling you that you have a hormone imbalance.

Gray and Red

An STD/STI may make your period smelly and cause it to appear as a mix of red and gray. This color of discharge, accompanied by pieces of gray tissue, can also occur if you are having a miscarriage, so see you doctor if this happens to you.

While it may not be the most pleasant thing to do, taking a moment to notice the color and consistency of your period blood is a great way to take note of your body's natural signals.[26]

SPOT CHECK

When your period leaks onto your undies, it is tempting to just fling them into the trash and buy a new pair, but even those ancient period panties with the overstretched elastic and the hole

---

BLOOD IN THE WATER

While most women are perfectly comfortable swimming in a pool even during their period, thanks to tampons and menstrual cups, those same women might think twice before swimming in the ocean because of a myth that sharks will smell the blood and come to eat you for lunch. However, not all species of shark are equally attracted to the smell of blood, but even for those drawn to it, like white sharks, scent alone often isn't enough to trigger a predatory response, especially from a distance. Sharks remain wary if they don't spot their regular, sure-thing prey, and they'd rather not take a chance on humans, no matter what the Sharknado franchise would like us to think.[27]

on the butt are worth saving and reusing because you are likely to leak in them again in a few months.

Learning how to get those stains out is almost as important as learning to always carry tampons or pads in your purse! The first thing to do is to give the offending panties a good cold-water rinse under the faucet as soon as you can, scrubbing them thoroughly with whatever soap is available—hand soap will do nicely—then launder them as usual. On light-colored underwear, you can try some hydrogen peroxide and then rinse thoroughly, but be warned that it may bleach out color on darker-colored panties. You can also check at the grocery or drugstore for a laundry or spot cleaner that is specifically formulated for blood. If it's your favorite pair of underwear, test to see if the spot remover will alter the color before you use it. These instructions work for bedsheets as well, because who hasn't woken up to that fun surprise of a leak or your period coming when you didn't expect it!

COPING WITH THE FLOW

Ever since women have walked the earth, we have had to come up with ways to manage our monthly visitor—ancient Romans are said to have fashioned their own tampons out of wool, Indonesian women are believed to have used vegetable fibers, and rolls of grass are said to have been used in parts of Africa. Hawaiian women used the "the furry part of a native fern," and ancient Japanese women made tampons from paper, securing them with bandages that they changed 10 to 12 times every day. But ever since 1933, when a Colorado doctor obtained a patent after he learned one of his female patients was inserting sponges each month, the game has changed. Leave it to a man to get a patent for something women have been using for centuries . . .[28]

When you stroll down the euphemistically named "feminine hygiene" aisle of your local drugstore or pharmacy today, you might home in on specifically what you are used to buying—probably something quite similar to what your mom bought you in your first years as a young woman. But if you take a minute to look around, you will notice myriad products to help you deal with your monthly flow that have been developed since the 1930s. A range of shapes, sizes, and materials are designed for light, medium, heavy, and overnight flow, and any number of brands are available in standard tampons and pads. There are even "sport" tampons and pads specifically sized for thongs. There are name-brand products in fancy boxes and there are store brands—both containing essentially the same items. There is also a range of lesser-known reusable menstrual products from the long-available menstrual cup to the new, and somewhat confusing to the newly initiated, fluid-absorbing underwear.

Despite the many variations on the theme, essentially your options for dealing with menstrual flow are tampons, pads, and menstrual cups, and what you use during your period comes down to personal preference. Some women prefer using a tampon for the convenience. Some women chose to use a pad because they are not comfortable with tampons. Some women use menstrual cups because they are reusable, reduce waste, and have less of a negative impact on landfills and the environment. Some women use different products at different times during their periods to deal with their level of flow or to use the products effectively. For example, someone who uses tampons during the day may use a pad at night because tampons are not recommended for overnight use. Or someone who uses a menstrual cup may back up that method with a pad or a panty liner. Whether you are set in your ways or ready for a change, it's

---

FREE THE TAMPON

Tampons can be liberating, but they can also be pretty dang expensive. Just think about it: If you buy a box of 36 tampons at the drugstore for $7 and use 4 per day for each of the 5 days of your period over a lifetime every month for the 42 years between the day you got your first period at 13 until menopause at 51, that's $1,773![29] And that's not including all of the pads, panty liners, Midol, emergency chocolate, and extra panties to replace the unsalvageable stained ones. But there is hope: A movement has begun to exempt tampons and other feminine hygiene products from sales tax (the "pink tax") because they are a health necessity. Repeat after us: Tampons are not a luxury item!

The Free the Tampons organization believes that tampons should be provided free of charge in schools, businesses, and public restrooms so that all women can have access to a necessity without cost or shame. Imagine that you get your period unexpectedly and you can have easy access to a pad or tampon. What a game changer! Visit them online at www.freethetampons.org.

certainly worth trying different products and different brands, because one company's product might not be right for you and another's will be the perfect fit.

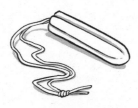

TAMPONS

Essentially a plug made of cotton or synthetic fibers (or a combination of both) that is inserted into the vagina, a tampon is used to absorb menstrual blood as it exits the cervix and prevents it from flowing out of the vagina. Tampons have a string for easy retrieval. Sometimes, because the string hangs outside of the body, it can get peed on when you go to the toilet, so some recommend changing your tampon every time you go to the bathroom. Either that or make sure that the string is safely to the side out of pee range. Seems like good advice—who wants a wet, urine-soaked string in their underwear? Ew.

Tampons come in a wide range of sizes and levels of absorbency. They also have different "delivery systems," too—in other words, some have applicators, some do not. Again, which type you use comes down to personal preference. Some women prefer using nonapplicator tampons because they feel that they can place the tampon more securely in their vagina when they guide it in with

---

MENSTRUATING MAIDENS

Even though tampons have been around in some form or another for as long as there have been periods, when they were first released onto the market as a commercially made product, the reactions ranged from skeptical to horrified. Many people were scandalized with the idea of women and girls touching their vulvas and vaginas and freaked out because they thought they might be feeling pleasure as a result of tampon insertions. There was a lot of discussion about the possibility of a tampon being able to break a hymen, resulting in the loss of virginity. People in the 1930s seem to have confused sex with the necessary practice of managing a woman's natural bodily functions—and unfortunately, some of these absurd ideas persist today.[30]

---

their finger. And with no applicator, there is less waste. Other women prefer using an applicator because they feel it is a better method of getting their tampon inserted properly. Some applicators are plastic; some are cardboard. Paper or plastic? Up to you!

Another option you may encounter is scented or deodorant tampons. These are best avoided, as they can lead to irritation and allergic reaction. Your vagina doesn't really need any help with odor control or to be infused with floral scents.

Because a tampon is internal, it can be more comfortable and convenient to use when doing sports, swimming, or other activities and can stop leaks before they happen. Tampons are easily portable and very convenient to use.

Some concerns have been raised about tampons as being

unhealthy and unsafe (see "Toxic Shock Syndrome (TSS)," below). If you choose to use tampons, no worries: The materials are typically natural, the bleaching process is toxin-free, and they are generally safe as long as you follow best practices guidelines on using them.

DOS

Do wash your hands before inserting your tampon.

Do change your tampon at least every 4 to 8 hours.

Do use a tampon that is right for your flow—smaller tampons for lighter days and larger tampons for heavier days.

Do remember to remove the last tampon you use during your

TOXIC SHOCK SYNDROME (TSS)

Toxic shock is a potentially life-threatening infection caused by bacteria called *Staphylococcus aureus*, more commonly known as "staph," or by *Streptococcus pyogenes* (group A strep).[31,32] It has been linked to superabsorbent tampons, leading to concern over using tampons in general. But if overblown stories in the media or anecdotes from a friend who had a friend who died from TSS have you considering swearing off tampons for good, keep in mind that if you change your tampon frequently, do not leave a tampon in overnight, and avoid superabsorbent tampons, you should not have a problem. If you are using tampons and you get a sudden fever, feel nauseated, vomit, and have a headache, you should get to your doctor to be checked out. Toxic shock is pretty rare—only 1 or 2 out of every 100,000 women will ever get it—and if you use your tampons correctly, you should be fine.[33]

period (you'd be surprised how many women forget) because it can cause an infection if left in too long.

DON'TS

Do not force a tampon when inserting—if you are having trouble, go to a smaller size.

Do not flush tampons down the toilet (wrap in toilet tissue and discard in the garbage).

Do not use a high-absorbency tampon if you don't need one (light days or between periods), as it can pull fluid from the vagina and damage the vaginal lining.

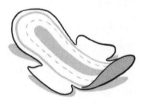

PADS

Also known as sanitary pads or sanitary napkins, some form of pad has been used by women to absorb blood from their periods for just as long as women have been experimenting with tampons. Before there were a thousand different types of pads and tampons filling an entire aisle, women had to either safety pin a pad to their underpants or—back before women wore the type of underpants we have today—wear a contraption called a sanitary belt. A bulky pad was attached to an adjustable belt and suspended between the legs to catch the flow. Leaks were a common occurrence, as the fluid often overwhelmed the pad. Just imagine running a 5K or rocking a pair of skinny jeans while wearing one of those!

And if you think a device like that should be relegated to the Middle Ages, remember that the adhesive pads we use today were not introduced until the 1970s.[34] Pads are so much higher tech both in their levels of absorbency and functionality nowadays, and they have been designed to fit all women, underwear styles, and preferences. Still, many women will choose not to wear their "best" underwear during their period not only to avoid stains but also to have underwear that can fully support a pad. Also because periods are weird, and you never know when even the most high-tech-sounding gel-absorption layer in your pad will fail you and you'll end up begging a stranger for a spare pad in a public restroom. Don't worry, it happens to the best of us!

There are a lot of choices when it comes to disposable pads. Some have absorbing gel, some are made of cellulose, some even have wings! Fun, right? Most pads are constructed so that the fluid is completely absorbed and that there is a layer of material between you and the absorbed blood so that your pubic hair and labia are not constantly wet and sticky. Despite how absorbent your pad is, it is a good idea to change it every 3 to 4 hours. It can be wrapped in toilet tissue and put in the trash, but never flushed.

Some pads have scents and deodorizers, which can irritate your labia. If you have skin allergies or if you are sensitive, read your packaging carefully and find unscented pads. Trust us, in all likelihood you smell just fine down there.

You can also get reusable pads that either attach to your underwear or use a special cloth panty liner where the pad is inserted into the panty liner. Reusable pads are washable, can be made of organic materials, and are largely free of plastics or chemicals. The upside is that they reduce your impact on the environment—there is no wrapper, no superabsorbent chemical materials going into landfills—and can cost less over time than buying disposable products each month. Some women feel that a downside to reusables is that you need to wash the pads, making them a bit more labor intensive. If you are at all uncomfortable dealing with blood, it can be a tough road to travel.

DOS

Do use the right pad for the right time in your cycle.

Do choose the type of pad that works best for you—disposable or reusable.

DON'TS

Do not use a pad for more than 3 to 4 hours.

Do not use overly perfumed pads, as they may cause irritation.

Do not flush pads; wrap in tissue and discard.

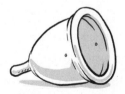

MENSTRUAL CUPS

Only recently beginning to rise in popularity, the original design for the menstrual cup—or "menstrual receptacle," as it was originally dubbed—was invented in 1884. The patent for the cup that we know and love today was awarded in 1937 to Leona Chalmers, an American actress and inventor.[35] Because the menstrual cup and the tampon were both invented and released commercially in the 1930s, why then did the tampon become a household item while the cup fell into obscurity—to be stocked only in small retailers like natural food stores—for almost 50 years? Well, in the first place, the original menstrual cup was made of latex—a material that was in short supply during World War II, which led to a stoppage in production. In the postwar years, competing with the established disposable market was an expensive proposition and cost these early companies too much money too fast.[36] So although this reusable product would have saved a lot of money and waste, the menstrual cup is a fairly recent addition to drugstore aisles.

A menstrual cup is a flexible rubber or silicone, well, cup that you insert into your vagina to catch the bloodflow during your period. Each brand is a little bit different in terms of size, material, and other features. They generally come in two sizes—one for women who have never given birth and one for those who have—and because they are flexible and the vagina stretches, you should be able to find one that works for you. One type of cup has a stem for ease in removal. Other cups are shaped more like a diaphragm and come in one size.

Cups are essentially like a reusable tampon; however, unlike tampons, they can stay in for up to 12 hours, so you don't have to worry about changing them frequently. They will give you the same benefits of using a tampon in that they are out of sight and will not interfere with any sports or activities. Not particularly high maintenance, menstrual cups require less care than disposable pads and tampons, and they only need a thorough washing every 12 hours. If you can't give it a full wash, rinse it, wipe it out with tissue, and give it a proper clean later. Some cups actually are disposable, either after one use or after your period is over.

On the downside, cups can leak, either when in place or when you remove them. So until you are familiar with how yours works for you, it might be a good idea to use a disposable or reusable pad or panty liner as backup—just in case.

A menstrual cup will take a little getting used to, both for inserting it to get it situated comfortably and taking it out without spilling blood when you remove it and pour the blood into the toilet. If you are icked out by the idea of handling containers of your period blood—as opposed to just dealing with it after it's absorbed into tampons or pads—cups may not be the right method for you. But there are a lot of pluses that may outweigh the slight ick factor. Women who use menstrual cups like the fact that they are eco-friendly, relatively low maintenance, don't expose you to any potential chemical irritants, and will cost less over time than using other products—most brands cost around $30 to $40. When you think about it, it is your blood, and it's coming out one way or another!

Because menstrual cups are inserted into your vagina, they do pose a risk for toxic shock (same as tampons,) but the risk is low. Mind your warning signs and get to a doctor if you have symptoms (see "Toxic Shock Syndrome (TSS)," page 64).

DOS

Do clean thoroughly every 12 hours while using.

Do clean extensively at the end of your period, either with special washes or by boiling for sterilization (see the manufacturer's instructions).

Do dispose of properly if you are using a disposable cup. No flushing; toss in the trash.

DON'TS

Do not leave in for more than 12 hours.

Do not panic if you have trouble removing the cup. Tensing up will make it more difficult. Practice, and patience, makes perfect.

MAIL-ORDER MENSTRUAL SUPPORT

If you find it inconvenient to get to the store to stock up on supplies or you don't want to get caught short, then you are in luck! A number of subscription services will deliver an assortment of supplies each month that you select to fit your needs. In addition to whatever pads or tampons you have ordered, most services will send some fun extras like lotions or herbal tea or Midol. Signing up for the monthly service can take the panic out of running out of supplies and give you something fun to look forward to that goes along with your period. Prices and products vary, so pop "period subscription box" into your favorite search engine and order away!

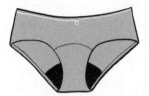

ABSORBENT PERIOD PANTIES

Made by an increasing number of companies and reaching a wider audience every day, period panties have gained market share over the past few years, giving way to stain-resistant, wicking, and absorbent workout clothes that have appeared on store shelves and online as well. While period panties may seem like a completely new innovation to many—and in many ways they are— experimentation in this area has been going on since the invention of so-called sanitary bloomers lined with rubber that predated even sanitary belts. Finally, fabric technology and smart design has advanced those unsanitary and unsightly original concepts into the sleek and practical solutions we have today.[37]

MENOPAUSE

"The Change" sounds pretty ominous doesn't it? Well, all women will get there eventually. And by "there," we mean menopause. You may have a slight detour through perimenopause—a time that can last anywhere from 2 to 8 years—but sooner or later, you will be menopausal.

Menopause is the time in life when hormone production decreases, the messages to your reproductive system slow down,

BLEEDING BEHIND BARS

On August 1, 2017, the Federal Bureau of Prisons released a memo that requires all federal prisons with female inmates to provide at least one brand of tampon, pad, and panty liner to prisoners for free. It seems shocking that these women didn't have these basic hygienic items previously, but there are recorded incidents of prison officers refusing to give women pads to punish them and of women trading sex for the supplies they needed. Of the many indignities that the 12,000 women in the United States incarcerated in federal facilities face—including giving birth while shackled down—this measure, if properly implemented and enforced, will go a long way toward respecting these women while they serve their time.[39]

and you will no longer get a period. Once you have stopped menstruating for a year, you are considered to be in menopause. The average age of menopause is around 51, but some reach menopause in their forties and some later than 51. Just as there is a range of ages when periods start, there is a range of ages when periods come to an end. The age at which your mom reached menopause can give you an indication for your own timing, but as with most things health and hormone related, your relative health and environment will definitely have an influence.

Before you start cheering for the end of periods as you know them, you should realize that it's not as if one month you have a period and the next you don't and then you are all done. There is a process, that varies from woman to woman, that takes you from actively menstruating to not menstruating at all. During perimenopause, you can experience skipped periods, late periods, heavy bleeding, or light bleeding. You can still get pregnant during this time of your life—however rarely.[38] Think about those moms in their late forties who have another baby right as their last kid started high school. Oops!

The symptoms that accompany perimenopause and menopause can be minimal, or some women are hit full force. Symptoms, which are very much linked to and triggered by hormones (or the lack thereof) include:

Cardiovascular disease

Depression

Dry vagina

Hot flashes

Irregular periods

Irritability

Osteoporosis

Sleep issues

Continuing to have your period is starting to sound better by comparison, right? The truth is that menopause, like menstruation, is a normal biological process. By being aware of symptoms, you can take measures to cope with them, roll with them, and take this change in your life in stride. Diet, exercise, lifestyle changes, and medications can ease symptoms. Maintaining a healthy diet, quitting smoking, and engaging in some form of exercise can all help with menopausal symptoms.

Because hot flashes can make you feel like you've been turned into a space heater, wearing layers of clothes that you easily remove if you become overheated can make a big difference. This also applies for at night, as many women get hit with flashes when sleeping, so use a couple of light covers instead of one heavy one so you can regulate how warm or cool you feel. Your partner is just going to have to get used to your nightly temperature adjustments or sleep on the couch!

Hormone replacement therapy (HRT) is an option that you can talk over with your health-care provider to see if it is something for you. Depending on the type of hormone, HRT can be delivered via pill, patch, cream, gel, or suppository. There are some risks associated with taking estrogen to combat menopausal symptoms, including heart disease, stroke, breast cancer, and blood clots, so be sure to weigh the pros and cons with your doctor.

Beyond HRT, some supplements like calcium and vitamin D can help with symptoms of bone loss associated with menopause as well as to help absorb calcium from food. Vaginal dryness can be countered with your favorite lube or with water-based vaginal moisturizers.

Menopause is just another stage of life where knowing what to expect can help you prepare and better cope with whatever comes your way.

Having your period can be nothing more than an inconvenience, or it can be a colossal pain, literally and figuratively. The good news is that there are multiple ways of coping with your period itself as well as any unwelcome emotional and physical symptoms that come along with that "time of the month." Remember—and we can't say this enough—that what is normal for you may be different for someone else, so rather than comparing with a friend or going to the Internet, be sure to check out any unusual symptoms with your doctor.

BIRTH CONTROL 101: PREVENTING PREGNANCY AND ENSURING SAFER SEX

WHETHER THE IDEA OF having a baby right this moment fills your belly with butterflies of anticipation or has your lunch threatening to make an encore appearance, it's just as important to know how to get pregnant as it is to know how not to. It may seem silly to go over it, but humor us as we flashback to "the Talk" you had with your mom on the edge of your bed or the section about "the birds and the bees" in that incredibly awkward health class. In your Anatomy 101 lesson, we covered the location of the various key players of your reproductive organs, but just as a little refresher, here's the lowdown.

Vagina: Where the penis goes in (if that's how you roll), ejaculates the sperm, and where the baby comes out

Ovaries: Where the egg matures and is released and is taken up by the fallopian tubes and delivered to the . . .

Uterus, aka the womb: Where if sperm meets egg, the fertilized egg implants in the uterine wall, and where the baby spends 9 months growing and getting ready to be born

There is a wide range of forms of birth control that are effective in preventing pregnancy and that you can choose from to suit your preferences and relationships. Birth control methods operate in various ways: They can regulate hormones to prevent ovulation (the Pill, patch, IUD), they can form a barrier to prevent the sperm from reaching an egg (condom, diaphragm, vaginal sponge), or they can stop ovulation (morning-after pill); some also kill sperm (spermicides). The best method for you is one that you will use regularly and correctly and that fits with your lifestyle as well as accommodates any health issues you may have. A birth control method that your friend thinks is perfect may not be the best for you, and vice versa. Weighing your options to address your individual needs may be best done with a healthcare provider so you can fully understand potential side effects that are linked to a particular birth control method, how the method works, the cost, and its effectiveness.

A BRIEF HISTORY OF BIRTH CONTROL

We've come a long way from inserting crocodile dung into the vagina like the ancient Egyptians used to do to prevent pregnancy. Currently, there is a huge range of birth control methods to suit every woman and lifestyle. The thanks for these multitude of options goes to modern science, but we would be remiss if we did not give a huge shout-out to birth control advocate Margaret Sanger for her push to make birth control accessible and *legal* for women. Yes, birth control for women used to be illegal. Fun times! Did we say that crocodile dung was an odd birth control method? Well, how about Lysol? (Yes, the same product used to disinfect the kitchen floor.) Believe it or not, women in the 1920s used Lysol to prevent pregnancy—not only was it an ineffective birth control method, it was pretty harsh on the lady parts.

Fast-forward to the 1960s and the invention of the birth control pill. The 1960s was also the time of the sexual revolution, and whether or not the Pill caused the sexual revolution by allowing women to engage in sexual activity without fear of pregnancy or if it was a by-product of the sexual revolution is up for debate. However, there is no debate about how many women embraced use of the Pill as a convenient, no-fuss method of birth control—it actually put birth control in their control. The 1990s saw medical and convenience advances like the birth control shot and emergency contraception. The 2000s added to effective birth control methods with vaginal rings, long-lasting intrauterine devices, skin patches, and hormone injections. In addition to these methods, there are over-the-counter products like spermicides (suppositories or foams) and the sponge, which (after some initial issues) is widely available over the counter. There are now extended-cycle birth control pills that use low doses of hormones to prevent a period from ever happening—and, of course, prevent pregnancy.[1]

Some birth control methods require a prescription; some are easily found in your local drugstore or pharmacy. Because of the variety of methods, it is worth having a conversation with your health-care provider or local clinic to assess which form of birth control is best for you and your lifestyle and so they can take into consideration any potential health issues or risks you may have. When you read the fine print on the packaging, you may see the range from perfect-use rate and the real-world rate. Because we don't live in a perfect world, we are going to give you the effectiveness rate—that is, how the product works when used the way most people use that particular method. Not perfectly, but much, much better than not using anything at all.[2]

THE MAN'S TURN

Although studies are in their early stages and researchers are working to perfect the hormone formula, women around the world are cautiously celebrating the soon-to-be-introduced birth control shot for men. After centuries of bearing the responsibility of not getting pregnant, it could be time for men to take a turn. And it doesn't seem like many women will too feel badly about the potential side effects men could experience: mood disorders, increased libido, acne, and muscle pain. Sound familiar? Despite those side effects, though, 75 percent of the clinical trial participants said that they would be willing to use this method.[3]

BIRTH CONTROL OPTIONS

Condoms are the oldest form of birth control, evidenced by cave paintings of "sheathed penises" that date all the way back to 15,000 BC. While we don't know what these ancient penises were sheathed with, there are records of ancient Romans wearing hand-sewn linen sheaths and evidence that, in the 1300s, Asian aristocrats were covering the tips of their penises with intestine, oiled paper, animal horns, and tortoise shells during sex. We wonder what 14th-century Asian aristocratic women thought about those animal horns . . .[4]

Happily, we have evolved beyond using animal horns when we get horny (see what we did there?), and technology has led to the development of birth control methods that are both unobtrusive and definitely more hygienic. That said, sometimes the tried-and-true methods are the go-to for most people. So, other than coitus interruptus, the condom is the oldest method in the bed, er, book.

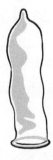

CONDOMS

Condom, rubber, French letter, raincoat, or johnny—no matter what you call it, it is the number one method for preventing pregnancy *and* preventing sexually transmitted diseases and infections. Okay, end of PSA.

Let's get some condom-related myths out of the way. A primary excuse for not wearing condoms is that doing so diminishes pleasure because the sex is not skin-to-skin, and some say that sex simply feels better without one. Well, lube can help with any friction issues, and there is a huge range of condoms that are thinner, coated with lube, flavored, studded and/or ribbed and with various bells and whistles that enhance pleasure both for him and for her. Let's just face it: You are going to be able to have a lot more sex if you get comfortable using condoms and your partners get comfortable as well—so bag it up!

Condoms are made of various materials: Latex, polyurethane, lambskin, and polyisoprene. Latex, polyurethane, and polyisoprene will all protect against sexually transmitted diseases or infections (STDs/STIs), whereas lambskin condoms (actually made from the intestinal membrane of a lamb) protect against pregnancy but are not effective against STDs and STIs. It has been said that one type of condom has a more natural feel than the others—usually the thinner the condom the better, the thinking goes—but you may love one type and feel unstimulated and uncomfortable with another. Experiment to see what works best. Be bold and try flavored condoms for oral or heat-activated condoms for some extra fun. And if you or your partner has a latex allergy, then you have choices that will not leave you with an allergic reaction in your genitals—because who wants that?

Another common myth is that condoms cause urinary tract infections (UTIs). The truth is that friction and irritation as well as bacteria can cause UTIs. In fact, using a condom can help keep bacteria out of the vagina as well as maintain the acidic pH of the vagina in balance. So don't blame the condom—just be sure you are have lots of pregame before you get busy.

Bottom line, the love glove is a great way to prevent pregnancy as well as to avoid STDs and STIs.

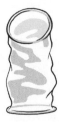

FEMALE CONDOM

The female condom is another hormone-free way to prevent both pregnancy and STDs and STIs, and it is 79 percent effective in doing so. Because it can be inserted several hours prior to sex, you don't have to have your passion interrupted while he wraps it up with a male condom or when you slip out of the sheets to put in a diaphragm or cervical cap.

The female condom is latex-free, made of nitrile (a flexible rubber), and does not contain any spermicides. It is essentially a long tube (about the same length as a condom but wider) that is closed at one end. There are flexible rings at each end; one at the closed end that anchors the female condom inside the vagina, and another at the other end that covers the opening to the vagina. It can take some getting used to, but it is another method of birth control that is effective, doesn't have to squash spontaneity, allows you to choose a birth control method that can be used in the moment, and can give you peace of mind that you are protected.

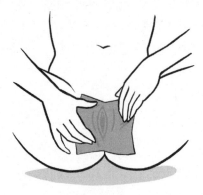

DENTAL DAMS

Used during cunnilingus, when your partner going down on your lady parts, or during analingus, when your partner going down on your back door, a dental dam is a rectangle of latex that is placed over the vulva or the anus to prevent the spread of STDs/STIs.

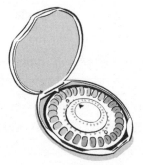

THE PILL

In 1957, when "the Pill" was first approved by the FDA not for birth control but for treatment of severe menstrual issues, an overwhelming amount of women very suddenly came down with some severe menstrual issues of their own and rushed to their doctor's office for a prescription.[5] And who can blame them? We can't imagine the constant worry that would accompany sex, the fear of dreams suddenly derailed by an unplanned pregnancy. To be set free from fear and to enjoy sex with a partner—things we take for granted these days—must have been such a relief for those women who popped those first little pills from their blister packs.

When used correctly—meaning taken at the same time each and every day like clockwork—birth control pills boast a 95 percent effectiveness rate—but when the unpredictable realities of life are considered, they are 92 percent effective. The most commonly prescribed pills are the so-called combination pills that contain a blend of estrogen and progesterone. They typically come in packs of 21 or 28. The pills deliver the dosage of hormones that will prevent you from ovulating: No ovulation = no egg, and no egg = no pregnancy. They increase mucus production so sperm has a more difficult time getting to the uterus and also thin the lining of the uterus so it is not receptive to implanting an egg should it become fertilized. You get your period when you stop taking the pills that contain hormones. So in a 28-day pack, the 7 remaining inactive placebo or sugar pills are there largely as a reminder to maintain the habit of taking a pill every day. If you are using a 21-day pack, you will not take a pill for 7 days, then you start your next pack. Because the creators of the Pill believed women would feel more comfortable if they continued to bleed each month, the 28-day menstrual cycle that you have while on hormonal contraception is artificial because it is triggered by the hormones in the pills, not by ovulation.[6]

The Pill is most effective if taken daily and at same time of day. You can set a reminder on your cell phone or take that day's pill when you brush your teeth in the morning or match taking it with any daily routine of your choice. The upsides of the Pill are that you will be protected from becoming pregnant (you don't have to say "hold that thought" when you want to have sex and go insert a diaphragm or other birth control method or fumble in the bedside drawer for a condom), it can alleviate some of the more painful aspects of menstruating, and you will know exactly when to expect your period each month. It takes the guesswork out of planning for supplies or surprises. But—and this is a big but—the Pill will not protect you from sexually transmitted diseases or infections.

Once you get into the habit, taking a daily pill is really no big deal. However, if you space and miss a day, you haven't necessarily blown it. Read the instructions that come with your prescription; most likely, if fewer than 24 hours have passed, you can just take the next pill and you should be fine. If you miss more than one day, then you can take two at a time and, to be on the safe side, use a backup birth control method like condoms or spermicide for a week. If you miss a few days, then you definitely need to use an alternate form of birth control and perhaps call your doctor to figure out the best next steps to see if you should continue with your current pack of pills or start a new pack.[7]

You can also use the combination pill to prevent your period from coming at all. Instead of taking the placebo pills, you would skip them and go straight into another pack of hormone pills. There is a potential for spotting if you follow this method for ceasing having a period, and you will need to speak with your doctor about your plans. To use your combination pills in this way, your prescription would need to be adjusted, since you will go through more packs of pills in a year than if you take the placebo pills and have a period each month.

The "Mini" Pill

This version of the Pill only contains the hormone progestin. The "mini pill" is commonly prescribed if you are breastfeeding or cannot take estrogen. Mini pills are a lot trickier if you miss a pill, because their effectiveness relies on a strict schedule—they need to be taken at the *same time* every day. If fewer than 3 hours have passed from your regular dosage time, and you remember (that alarm on your smartphone is begging to be used!), take that skipped pill right away and take the next one 24 hours later. To be on the safe side, use another form of birth control for the next couple of days. The timing issue with mini pills can make them a bit more challenging to cope with; it is a good idea to read the insert information that comes with your pills so you can use them correctly and effectively. A call to your doc or clinic for clarification couldn't hurt if you are confused about taking the Pill or if your schedule has been messed up.

The mini pill is slightly less effective than the combination pill, but if you can't deal with estrogen or are breastfeeding, it is the right way to go. However, if you have a crazy schedule and aren't able to take your mini pills on a regular basis, another form of birth control might be better for you.

Extended-Cycle Birth Control Pills

Because why have more periods than you need to (see "Do You *Need* to Get a Period?"), another form of birth control pill limits the number of times per year that you will get your period. Extended-cycle birth control pills contain a combination of ethinyl estradiol and levonorgestrel so they prevent ovulation and make the cervical mucus a thicker barrier to sperm. When you are prescribed extended-cycle birth control pills, you will take an "active" pill daily for 84 days (12 weeks) followed by a week off to get your period, when you would take the "inactive"

DO YOU *NEED* TO GET A PERIOD?

"I love getting my period." Said no one, ever. Let's face it: Nobody really enjoys having a period—so why not just stop it entirely? A period is not a medical necessity, so you can go ahead and postpone your visits from Aunt Flo. With some new birth control pills, this is a real possibility. If you use this type of birth control, you will never menstruate until you stop taking the pills. These specific pills stop ovulation, so the lining in the uterus doesn't build up, although you may have light bleeding that technically isn't a period.[8]

Another thing: It is a misconception that your period somehow cleans your body and your uterus. Having a period has nothing to do with cleaning and is all about getting rid of something your body doesn't need. If there is no baby, there is no need for the uterine lining.

pills to remind you to maintain the daily habit of taking a pill. Under this regimen, you will get only four periods a year, where with the standard combination pill, you get one each month. There is even an extended birth control method that you can take every day and you never get a period—until you stop taking the pills.

If you miss an extended-cycle pill, take two the next day and then take one per day until you finish the pack. When you start extended-cycle birth control pills, you can experience break-through bleeding, but this should resolve once you have been taking them for a few months.

Side Effects of the Pill

Because all forms of the Pill are made of hormones, and we know how hormones can wreak havoc on your body, it should come as no surprise that the Pill has some side effects that are remarkably similar to the physical and emotional aspects of having a period. Do weight gain, spotting, breast tenderness, headaches, and moodiness sound familiar? When you first start the Pill, you may experience some of these side effects. But before you quit, it's worth giving it time to see if the issues resolve on their own. It can take about 3 months for your body to adjust to the synthetic hormones of the Pill. There have been some reported links between birth control and depression, but studies are not conclusive.[9] As always, if an issue persists and seems out of the ordinary, consult with your doctor, as there are many different combinations of hormones and formulas that will work better for you.

THE PILL . . . IT'S NOT JUST FOR PREVENTING PREGNANCY

Because it delivers a steady does of hormones, the birth control pill can be helpful in treating hormonally triggered issues like menstrual irregularity, heavy bleeding during periods, cramps, migraines, acne, endometriosis, and polycystic ovary syndrome (PCOS). If you have any of these conditions, your doctor may prescribe the Pill for you. You may also be prescribed birth control pills if you are taking a medication that—should you become pregnant—would be harmful to a developing baby. For example, if you are prescribed isotretinoin (Accutane) for severe acne, you are required to pledge to use birth control, and often the Pill is the first choice.[11]

Certain side effects that can accompany the Pill are not common but can be serious and should send you directly to your doctor or the ER. An easy way to remember these bad boys is ACHES.

A—Abdominal (stomach) pain

C—Chest pain

H—Headache (severe)

E—Eye problems (blurry vision)

S—Swelling or aching in the thighs and legs[10]

Keep in mind that the Pill is a prescription medication, so if you are going to a doctor other than your ob-gyn for any other health issue or treatment, be sure to mention that you are on the Pill. Some medications, particularly specific antibiotics, can reduce the effectiveness of the Pill, and you'll want to call in some backup for pregnancy prevention.

The Pill is not for you if you smoke (especially if you are over age 35), have high blood pressure, have heart disease, have breast or uterine cancer, or have had, or are subject to, blood clots.

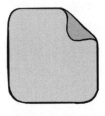

SKIN PATCH

If taking a daily pill is too high maintenance for you, then the patch may be a better option. The patch—about 92 percent effective—can be obtained by prescription from your doctor. Named one of the Best Innovations of 2002 by *Time* magazine,[12] the patch is like a square Band-Aid or sticker that adheres to your body and delivers hormones similar to those in the Pill into your system through your skin. There are three patches in a 28-day cycle, and it's important to apply your new patch around the same time each week. The week you don't use a patch will be when you get a period.

The patch adheres directly to clean, dry skin (no makeup or lotions or powders should go near or under the patch) and can be applied to the upper arm, belly, buttocks, or upper back. You should not apply it to your breasts, because the hormones can directly affect the breast tissue. It needs to go somewhere on your body where it will be in direct, constant contact with your skin and where it will not get rubbed, which may cause it to fall off. Avoid placing it near a bra strap or where the band of your underwear might catch on it. You can place it on your body where it will be covered by clothes, but if you are naked, it's going to be out there for your partner to see (or a larger audience, depending on how you roll). Plus, depending on your skin color, a beige square may not be invisible on your skin anyway. Once you stick it on, you can largely forget it—you can swim, shower, and exercise with the patch on. It's a good idea to check throughout the week to be sure it remains firmly stuck to your skin. If it comes loose or falls off, you should contact your doctor.

Because of the hormone content of the patch, the side effects are similar to the majority of hormone treatments, but you also run the risk of skin irritation where it has been stuck to your body. Switching where you place the patch from week to week can keep your skin irritation to a minimum. If you have sensitive skin, the patch may not be right for you.

As with all medications, let your health-care providers know you are using the patch, as there may be medications that negatively interact with the hormones in the patch, in which case you'll want to seek out alternatives.

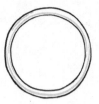

VAGINAL RINGS

This form of prescription birth control brings a whole new meaning to the phrase "Put a ring on it!" Vaginal rings are about 2 inches in diameter, clear, and contain a combination of hormones much like the combination pill. The big difference is that the ring is inserted into the vagina like a tampon, and the hormones are slowly released to prevent ovulation, thicken cervical mucus, and potentially prevent a fertilized egg from implanting in your uterus. The ring is inserted once a month and left in for 3 weeks. At the end of week 3, you remove it, and then you get your period. Because it is a once-a-month birth control, you don't have to deal with daily reminders, and a plus is that the ring can be worn during exercise or sex. It is also about 92 percent effective for most users.

The side effects are similar to those of the combination pill in terms of cardiovascular issues like blood clots, heart attacks, and stroke. Because the ring is inserted in your vagina and stays there for 3 weeks, there is a risk for vaginitis, irritation, or discharge. If you think your discharge or irritation has blossomed into an infection, see your doctor. As a rule, any unusual discharge should be brought to your doctor's attention.

Rings can sometimes become dislodged during sex or even during a bowel movement. If this happens, you can rinse it off and reinsert it. As long as you reinsert it within 3 hours of its coming out of your vagina, your pregnancy protection will remain firmly in place.

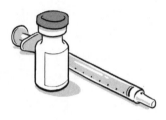

THE SHOT

If the patch falls in the category of "fix it and forget it," at least for a week, Depo-Provera, aka the birth control shot, is a longer-lasting option that, if you don't mind shots, can be great for you. The shot contains progestin (just like the mini pill) and has similar side effects. The upshot (ha!) is that you only need an injection every 12 weeks, delivered into your upper arm or butt by your doctor. So you don't have to think about your birth control daily or weekly, but only every few months. It is also about 97 percent effective as long as you get the shots on a regular schedule.

The shot can be used while breastfeeding, it can be appropriate for women who can't take a combined pill, and it can deliver the benefits of the Pill (in addition to birth control), including helping resolve heavy periods. Because of its lasting effects in the body, the hormones linger for some time in your system even after you stop getting the shots. The hormone in the injec-

THE DARK HISTORY OF THE SHOT

While the invention of the birth control shot has been freeing for many women, it's impossible to hide from the deeply unsettling baggage that accompanies it. In the 1960s and 1970s, the clinical trials for Depo-Provera were conducted mostly on black, rural, and/or low-income women, and women in developing nations—in many cases without their consent or knowledge. Sadly, this occurrence is not a unique one and, when the FDA approved the shot in 1992, the National Women's Health Network made its objections known. Now, even though over one million people benefit from this innovation, it's essential to look back and learn from this unforgivable history and make sure this type of duplicitous, racist, and classist clinical trial is never again repeated.[13]

tion stops ovulation, and that may not resume for several months after you no longer receive the shots, during which time you will still need a form of birth control. It is common for your period to stop when you are on the shots because the hormones interfere with the production of the lining of the uterus and there is no tissue or blood to shed each month. On the other hand, you can also experience spotting or bleeding while on the shot, but it is most often minimal. If the spotting or bleeding becomes an issue, speak with your doctor, and she can discuss alternatives with you.

You should not have the shot if you have hepatitis, recently had cancer, or suffer from osteoporosis. Be sure to discuss your health history with your doctor before deciding on this method of birth control.

THE IMPLANT

What if we told you there was a birth control method that would last for years, where nothing has to be placed in your lady parts and you didn't have to worry about getting pregnant? No, we're not talking about abstinence or taking a vow of chastity or secluding yourself in a cave—there is another way! The implant is a form of birth control that is totally hands-off because it is inserted under the skin in your arm. Sounds like it's right out of the plot for a science fiction film, doesn't it? No worries, it's a common form of birth control that is 99 percent effective and unobtrusive. Only you and your doctor need to know that the implant is there. It just takes a couple of minutes for your doctor to insert the small plastic rod, about the size of a toothpick, into the inside of your upper arm. The rod contains a hormone called etonogestrel, and it's a form of progestin. If that name sounds familiar, know that the cast of hormone characters called on to prevent pregnancy is not large. You will remember that progestin is in the mini pill as well as in the patch and the shot.

The implant in your arm releases the hormone over time and works to stop ovulation. The implant is in for the long haul and can prevent pregnancy for up to 3 years. While they have an implant, some women can stop bleeding altogether or have slightly altered bleeding patterns. The side effects of the implant are similar to those of other hormonal birth control methods and include weight gain, spotting, mood changes, and troubled skin. They can be handled just as you would the side effects from any other method of birth control.[14]

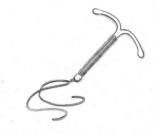

IUD—INTRAUTERINE DEVICE

An intrauterine device—or IUD—is a long-term form of birth control that is inserted directly into your uterus by your doctor. It is the ultimate in "out of sight, out of mind" birth control., Based on typical use, IUDs are 45 times more effective that the Pill and 90 times more effective than male condoms.[15] Although IUDs have had a bit of a bad rap from a 1970s version called the Dalkon Shield (sounds like something out of *Star Wars*, doesn't it?) that led to a high incidence of infection for the women using it, IUDs today have a much better record. According to the Centers for Disease Control and Prevention, IUDs are becoming more popular than ever: 4.4 million women had one in 2015![16]

An IUD is a flexible, plastic, T-shaped device that has a string attached to it for removal by your doctor. The arms of the T flex for insertion and removal. It is about half the size of a tube of lip balm, but because it goes into your uterus, a doctor is required to insert the device to get it placed accurately. She will do so through a simple procedure that can be a bit uncomfortable—some women get cramps and some spotting immediately after insertion—but is not a huge deal. An over-the-counter pain medication can usually do the trick to deal with any discomfort. IUDs are pretty low maintenance—you only have to check periodically that the string for retrieval is still in place—and they have manageable side effects. Despite what you might have heard, you do not have to have been pregnant or have delivered a baby to be able to use an IUD.

There are two types of IUDs: The hormone-based form has an effect on ovulation, and the nonhormonal copper version uses copper's properties as a natural spermicide to create an unfriendly environment for any sperm in the area.

Hormone-Based IUDs

Hormone-based IUDs contain forms of progestin and work by thickening the mucus in the cervix, as well as by making the lining of the uterus thinner and nonreceptive to an embryo implanting, and some prevent ovulation. Brands vary in size. They can remain in your uterus and continue to provide protection from pregnancy from 3 to 6 years, again, depending on the type you and your doctor choose.

Copper-Based IUDs

Copper-based IUDs are also made of flexible plastic, but instead of using hormones, they rely on the spermicidal properties of copper to prevent the sperm from getting to an egg. Sperm do not like copper, and this can come in handy if you find yourself in a situation where you have had unprotected sex or the condom broke, because copper-based IUDs can be used as a form of emergency contraception as long as you can get a quick appointment scheduled. If you have a copper IUD inserted within 5 days of having unprotected sex, it can effectively kill the sperm and prevent pregnancy. Then you can leave the IUD in and have protection for years to come. Copper-based IUDs can provide protection for up to 12 (!) years.[17]

The retrieval string on an IUD, which is made of a thin plastic, extends through your cervix into your vagina. The string softens over time, but if your partner can feel the string during sexual intercourse, speak with your doctor, as it may be possible to trim the string and still have the IUD removed easily by a doctor when you want to. Most women find that the string eventually tucks itself beside the cervix, out of the way of sex and tampons.

The side effects of IUDs are rarely a major hassle and can last for about 3 months as your body gets used to having the IUD seated in your uterus. Side effects can include, pain, backache, spotting, heavy bleeding, and irregular periods. The copper-based IUD is more likely to give you heavier periods and worse menstrual cramps. As always, if pain or discomfort increase or you just can't deal with the side effects, talk to your doctor to be sure all is well.

IUDs are not permanent—even though they might seem like they are when you have 3 to 12 stress-free years stretching out ahead of you—and can be removed, by your doctor, at any time. So if you no longer want an IUD or if you decide that you want to become pregnant, it can be taken out.

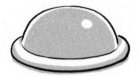

DIAPHRAGM AND CERVICAL CAP

While less common in recent years, these reusable, sperm-blocking methods of birth control that you insert yourself are available for prescription from your doctor. They come in different sizes; your ob-gyn will measure and prescribe the correct size for you. They work by covering the entrance to your cervix so sperm cannot move from your vagina to the uterus and fertilize an egg.

The primary difference between the diaphragm and the cap is size: The diaphragm is larger, and the cap, which is smaller, fits snugly over the cervix. The diaphragm is a silicone dome with a flexible base that you insert into your vagina, and it blocks the entrance to the cervix. The cervical cap is shaped like a thimble and a bit more precisely placed on the surface of the cervix.

To doubly ensure that no sperm survives its time in the vagina and goes where it shouldn't, these pregnancy preventers must be used with spermicide (nonhormonal foams, creams, gels—your choice).

Some troubleshooting tips: Before using your diaphragm or cervical cap, check for any tears or holes, as they will significantly reduce effectiveness for obvious reasons. Sometimes a cap or diaphragm can slip or dislodge during intercourse. They

WEIGHT GAIN AND BIRTH CONTROL

A common complaint about birth control is that it causes weight gain, but because your naturally occurring hormones may react with the synthetic hormones of birth control, it is hard to know in advance if one particular form of birth control will cause *you* to gain weight. With estrogen-based birth control, the weight gain is often due to retaining water. Some birth control pills contain a diuretic so that basically you will pee out any additional water weight. If the birth control you are using does not contain estrogen, then the weight gain you experience may be in the form of fat. This is most common with birth control shots. If you gain weight while on the Pill or other birth control, speak with your doctor. You may be able to counter the weight gain with changes in diet and exercise, or you may want to explore a different form of birth control.[18]

can be tricky to remove easily. It can take time getting used to inserting and taking them out. If you are having trouble, or are not sure how to know when the device is inserted properly, check with your doctor, and she can demonstrate for you.

You insert the device prior to having intercourse. (Every. Single. Time.) You can plan ahead, because they can be inserted up to 6 hours before sex and need to remain in place for 6 hours after. Don't leave a diaphragm in for more than 24 hours or more than 48 hours for the cervical cap.

Typically, these devices do not interfere with sex, except for the part where, if you hadn't already done so already, you need to excuse yourself and take time to insert them. Sometimes they can become dislodged in various positions or with vigorous thrusting. They don't have the side effects associated with hormonal-based birth control methods and don't impact your cycle or fertility. You will get your period the way you normally do. If you typically use a diaphragm or cap as birth control and then want to get pregnant, all you need to do is not use it. A diaphragm has a slightly higher effectiveness rate than the cervical cap, and the cap may be better for use by women who have not yet had children. They are effective around 84 percent of the time. The exception is if you are a woman who has had children and who uses the cervical cap—the effectiveness rate is about 68 percent in that case.

Some side effects of these methods can include urinary tract infections or irritation due to latex or spermicide sensitivity or allergy. Having lots of UTIs, vaginal irritation, or a weird rash and you have been using a diaphragm or cap? Then speak with your doctor. A simple switch of spermicide may do the trick, or you may need to consider another method of birth control.

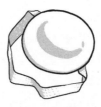

THE SPONGE

Over the counter and available without a prescription, another form of sperm-blocking birth control that you can insert before having intercourse is the sponge. This is a round, spermi-cide-filled foam device with a retrieval loop that is, well, spongy. You insert it in your vagina up to 24 hours before having sex. Like the diaphragm or cervical cap, because it is placed deep in your vagina, neither you nor your partner should be able to feel it during intercourse. You need to leave it in for at least 6 hours after the last time you have sex. You don't take it out and rein-sert it, because it is one-time use only—although in the plus col-umn, you can use it multiple times during one sex session, and you toss it in the trash when done.

You don't need a prescription, it's portable, and it doesn't do anything to your cycle or influence hormones, which is a major reason why some women use it. The effectiveness rate varies with usage, 68 to 84 percent, and it is more effective for women who have not given birth. It should not remain inside you for more than 30 hours. There is a risk for TSS (see page 64) with the sponge. If you are sensitive to spermicides,

---

SPONGE WORTHY

In the 1980s, the sponge was hugely popular, and then the device hit a snag in production, causing it to be unavailable. Many women were upset because they liked the ease of use, the no hormones, and the fact women were in control of birth control. The popularity led to an episode of *Seinfeld* where the character Elaine was stockpiling the sponge and only getting busy with partners who were "sponge worthy." I am sure that Elaine would be thrilled with the resurgence in popularity of her favorite birth control method!

polyurethane, or sulfa drugs, the sponge might not be for you. Also, it can irritate the vagina, and because you need to add water to activate the spermicide, some women say it makes sex "messier." You can't use it when you are on your period or bleeding for any reason.

EMERGENCY CONTRACEPTION

If you have had unprotected sex or had what is commonly referred to as a "birth control failure" (the condom broke, or you realized you haven't taken your birth control pills for a couple of days), then you may need to seek a form of emergency contraception. Emergency contraception stops a pregnancy before it can start, and although it's not ideal, it's essential if you do not want to become pregnant.

As mentioned on page 97, a copper IUD can be used as emergency contraception as long as it is inserted in your uterus by your doctor within 5 days of unprotected sexual intercourse. Then it can stay in to continue to provide you with pregnancy protection until you are ready to have it removed. But hormone-based emergency contraception, also commonly known as "the morning-after Pill," is available by prescription as well as over the counter. If you are seeking emergency contraction, check your state's laws; some states allow pharmacists to refuse to dispense emergency contraception. You may also be able to purchase emergency contraception online: For Ella, go www.ella-kwikmed.com, and for AfterPill, go to http://afterpill.com.

Over-the-counter emergency contraception contains the hormone levonorgestrel (a progestin) and comes in one-pill or two-pill dosages depending on the brand. It is effective when taken within 3 days or 72 hours of your bedroom slipup. Another type that you can take up to 5 days from having unprotected sex contains ulipristal acetate and is available by prescription only, but the pills work to delay or inhibit ovulation, which is why they are time sensitive. If you are already pregnant, they will not work.

These pills are not intended to be used regularly for birth control—break out these pills in case of *emergency* only! They have side effects like nausea, dizziness, and headache and can cause changes in your cycle, such as giving you earlier, later, or a heavy period in the same month when you have taken the emergency birth control, so they aren't something you want to take regularly anyway.[19, 20]

Although it might be awkward to ask a pharmacist for one of these emergency options, remember that it's their job to dispense them to you and it's your body and your right to get what you need. Even if you have to buy a bunch of items to hide the box from other shoppers, don't delay or get intimidated, because the clock starts ticking the moment of the mistake and it's up to you and your partner to quickly decide on a solution

MYTHS ABOUT EMERGENCY CONTRACEPTION PILLS (ECPS)

There is no room for old wives' tales when you are talking about emergency contraception. Here are a few of the myths you might hear and the facts you need to remember about emergency contraceptive pills (ECPs).

Myth: They cause abortions.

Fact: Levonorgestrel, the progestin hormone in most ECPs, prevents pregnancy by delaying ovulation and has no effect on a pregnancy. ECPs are not the same as a medical abortion.

Myth: Drinking and taking drugs the night before makes taking an ECP dangerous.

Fact: Not true—alcohol, cigarettes, and drugs the night before have no impact.

Myth: If I take an ECP today, I can have unprotected sex tomorrow risk-free.

Fact: ECPs are a one-time deal. The way they

and confidently follow through. And make sure you go dutch and split the cost with your partner, if possible!

ABORTIONS

Performed when there is an unplanned pregnancy, when it is determined that a fetus is not viable, or when the woman's health or life is at risk, an abortion is a process that terminates work actually puts you at higher risk of pregnancy soon after, because ovulation is only blocked for a few days, and if more sperm finds its way into the fallopian tubes and is there waiting when an egg is released, there is that much more of a chance the egg will be fertilized.

Myth: ECPs can mess with your fertility in the long term if you take them too frequently.

Fact: This is a baseless claim. Because ECPs prevent about seven out of eight pregnancies that would otherwise occur, they are actually less effective than other types of birth control like the Pill, patch, and ring and much less effective than the IUD or implant. Remember: ECPs are for emergencies for which you aren't prepared. Be familiar with these methods should an emergency arise, but find a method of birth control that works for you and that you will use consistently. That's your best defense.[21]

a pregnancy. While just under a century ago, in the late 1920s, some 15,000 women a year died from complications related to abortions, the procedure—when a patient has access to it—is now very safe and relatively painless.[22]

Roe v. Wade was a landmark decision made by the US Supreme Court in 1973 that made abortion legal in the United States. Ever since, there have been protests, challenges, and legislation passed that seek to limit women's access to abortion. For decades, pro-life and pro-choice proponents have clashed over this hotly contested and deeply personal issue—not just on the streets in front of clinics where they can be seen, but in state houses and in the White House—and there doesn't seem to be an end in sight to the battle over what is often framed as the fetus's or baby's right to life versus the woman's right to choose what happens to her own body.[23] As a result of this legislative tug-of-war over women's bodies, although the procedure is currently legal in the United States, over 80 percent of counties have no abortion providers, and some whole states have only one or two. While upholding *Roe v. Wade* with one hand, the US Supreme Court has used the other hand to allow states to erect barriers to abortion through denying public funds to pay for the abortions of poor women and enacting parental consent and notification requirements, mandatory waiting periods, and "counseling sessions" that often provide misinformation about abortions themselves, the inherent risks, and subsequent issues with fertility and health.

In her book *When Abortion Was a Crime*, Leslie J. Reagan suggests that abortion has always been an ideological struggle more than a scientific one, a legal one, or a religious one.[24] How free should women be to have sex without being required to submit to pregnancy and motherhood? How much of a right to a life outside of that traditional wife/mother role should she be allowed? As our country continues to have this seemingly unending debate, it's important that we know the rights we have and how we can exercise them now to keep ourselves healthy and our voices part of the conversation. A good resource to check for information is the Guttmacher Institute, at www

.guttmacher.org/state-policy/explore/overview-abortion-laws, for an overview of laws and a breakdown of state-by-state regulations that may impact you.[25]

Let's walk you through the abortion process. First things first—and this might seem painfully obvious—you need to take a pregnancy test. Not all missed periods mean you are pregnant, and the only way to really know is to take a test and then have the pregnancy confirmed by a doctor or medical professional. It's not like in a romance novel when someone just suddenly knows she is pregnant—the test is a vital first step in confirming your situation. Only then will you be in a position to weigh your options and decide what is best for you: parenthood, adoption assistance, or abortion. Each choice is valid and there for your consideration, and it's your choice to make.

If you choose to have an abortion, there are two avenues to terminating a pregnancy: medical and surgical.

Medical

The so-called abortion pill, otherwise known as RU-486, which was approved by the Food and Drug Administration in 2000, is referred to as a medical abortion and it is available to women during the first 10 weeks of pregnancy. According to the Centers for Disease Control and Prevention, as of 2013 (the most recent data available[26]), about 20 percent of abortions were medical, during which the women took the abortion pill or— more accurately—abortion pills. In reality the "abortion pill" is not really a single pill at all but two pills that contain different hormones and that are taken at different times. The first is a hormone that disrupts the environment in the uterus—the hormone mifepristone works against progesterone, which is the hormone that encourages the uterus to allow the fetus to grow—and the second pill, taken 24 to 48 hours after the first pill, contains the hormone misoprostol, which causes contractions that work to cause you to miscarry. The pill causes bleeding and cramping, and the experience is similar to what happens during a miscarriage. You can have heavy bleeding, cramping, nausea, and headache. If any of these symptoms becomes severe, seek medical attention.

The abortion pill is available across the United States, but some states have restrictions on how and from whom you can get a prescription or if you have to take the medication in a doctor's office. As we mentioned before in the box about myths surrounding emergency contraceptive pills: The abortion pill is *not the same* as the morning-after pill. The morning-after pill prevents a pregnancy from being established; the abortion pill aborts a pregnancy that is in its early stage.

Surgical

If a woman is beyond 10 weeks and wishes to terminate her pregnancy, then she will need to have a surgical abortion, although she could have chosen to surgically terminate before 10 weeks. In most states, you have up to 14 weeks after your last period to have a surgical abortion, because terminating a pregnancy in the late second trimester or in the third trimester is illegal in many states. Exceptions exist for abortions in the third trimester that are deemed medically necessary, such as a situation of a severe birth defect and a mother's health in danger. Although the law in the United States gives women the right to obtain an abortion, a woman can't just seek one out at any stage in her pregnancy. She needs to act quickly so that she can safely and legally explore all of her choices and not be left in a situation without options.

You can have a surgical abortion at a clinic or doctor's office. If you go to a clinic, you may well find yourself confronted by those who are protesting against abortion. They may bar your entrance to the building and attempt to shame you. Posing as a friendly concerned citizen, they may give you misinformation about where you can get care. They may just shout and wave signs. While it may be difficult to get through this gauntlet, many clinics have volunteers or staff who can escort you into the clinic, where you can have full access to the care you are entitled to.

If you are not under the care of a private physician, you can find information about clinics via Planned Parenthood and the National Abortion Federation (see Resources for contact information), where they list reputable abortion clinics to ensure you receive quality care. Rules and regulations vary greatly from state to state, and you may need to be given certain government-required information and then come back another day. Some states have a waiting period between the time you come in seeking an abortion and when you can have the procedure.

Because procedures and regulations vary from provider to provider and state to state, what follows are general guidelines on what you can expect should you choose to have an abortion.

Prior to the procedure, you will likely be asked about your medical history, have blood tests and a urine test to confirm your pregnancy, and perhaps be given an ultrasound to see how far along you are. You will most likely receive information about your options as well as an explanation about what will happen during the procedure.

During one method, suction or "vacuum aspiration" is used to remove the tissue from the uterus. You will be given pain meds and probably light sedation, after which a speculum is inserted into your vagina, the opening of the cervix is dilated, and a small suction tube is inserted through the cervix into the uterus. After the procedure, you will likely have cramping and bleeding, and you will be given instructions by the clinic or doctor on how to care for yourself, which may include a prescription for antibiotics as well as being told not to have sex for at least a week or two and to be sure to use birth control when you resume having sex. There is a risk for infection of the cervix and uterus following an abortion, so you don't want to put anything in your vagina—even tampons—until you are completely healed.

If you are over 14 weeks pregnant and up to 24 weeks, you will need to have a procedure known as a D&C, which stands for "dilation and curettage," or D&E, which is "dilatation and evacuation." The cervix needs to be dilated for the procedure, and because it can take some time to open, you may be given medication to open the cervix or your doctor will insert dilators into your cervix. Either way, it will take some hours or even overnight before your cervix is opened enough for the full D&C. When you are ready and the cervix has dilated sufficiently, you will be given pain medication as well as mild sedation/anesthesia. Tools are used to remove tissue from inside the uterus. Finally, suction is applied to make sure all tissue has been removed. Following an abortion, you may have cramping or bleeding. An over-the-counter pain reliever will usually be adequate to deal with any pain. Abortions are low-risk, safe medical procedures and do not impact future fertility—unless there are complications or you subsequently develop an infection, both of which are uncommon. If you develop a fever, are bleeding excessively, have severe abdominal pain that won't go away, or are generally feeling sick, then you should contact your doctor or clinic.

PREGNANCY

Okay, so remember the beginning of the chapter when we gave you an adult version of "the Talk" and then told you about all the ways not to end up with a baby? Well, here's the flip side. There are a wealth of books devoted to the how and what of getting pregnant and being pregnant, so we'll just cover some of the basics here and get to what happens to your vagina during pregnancy in and after childbirth.

WHAT TO EXPECT

As with all things related to your reproductive system, hormones play a huge role in what happens to your body and how you feel during pregnancy. Myths abound when it comes to pregnancy, and the one that really sets women up for feeling bad about themselves is "You'll love it!" And "You'll glow!" Sure, some women will rock that serene Madonna momma-to-be look, but others only shine with sweat as they navigate the world with a basketball-size belly and unpredictable hormones, or they'll have "morning sickness" all day long. Just remember that feeling badly or not enjoying your pregnancy doesn't mean that you don't want to be pregnant or that you won't be a good mom. You have our official permission to wish you could see your feet and crave whatever strange food combination your pregnant brain has concocted for you this week.

No matter how you feel while pregnant, and everyone has her own experience, certain issues commonly arise. Because of changes in hormones, vaginal discharge is very common during pregnancy, and you can be more susceptible to vaginal or yeast infections (see pages 200–202 for more information). Typical discharge is thin and white—a little like uncooked egg whites. If you notice an odor or itch, talk to your doctor. There are easy ways to treat vaginal or yeast infections, even when you are pregnant, using over-the-counter suppositories as well as natural remedies—just check with your doctor first before you self-diagnose. During pregnancy you can also be prone to urinary tract infections (UTIs; see pages 222–224). One of the symptoms of a UTI is that you feel like you need to pee more often—and guess what? That also happens when you are pregnant. So you should watch for the other signs of a UTI, like strong-smelling urine or a burning sensation when you pee, and let your ob-gyn know.

Because of increased blood volume and flow throughout your body, your vagina can become swollen and potentially a bit more sensitive—hey, we didn't say it was all bad! You may have light bleeding or spotting at different times during your pregnancy, and while that can be perfectly normal, you'll want to touch base with your health-care provider about any unusual bleeding—even if the spotting or bleeding stops. If you have severe cramping along with bleeding, then call immediately.

The appearance and scent of your vulva and vagina can change during pregnancy, too. You may not be able to see this one without a mirror, but one rather interesting change is that your labia and vulva may take on a tinge of blue color because of increased bloodflow and blood vessels. You might also develop varicose veins in your vulva, which can cause swelling and discomfort but will usually go away several weeks after delivery. The scent and taste of your vaginal secretions may change because of hormones and the relative acidity of your discharge, so if your partner comments about the change, just explain that it's temporary and all will return to normal hue, taste, and smell after you deliver.[27]

SPECIAL DELIVERY

We've mentioned previously that the vagina is very flexible and has lots of folds and bumps to stretch and accommodate all shapes and sizes of penises and sex toys. Well, the ultimate in stretching happens during delivery. During birth, contractions push the baby so that it travels from the uterus, through the cervix, into the birth canal (aka vaginal canal), and it exits through the opening to the vagina. Everything stretches! You are pretty much a superhero down there, and you probably haven't even given it much thought!

Also, it really hurts. Like, it really, really hurts. But it's totally worth it.

Through incredible advances in modern technology, there are machines where men can now experience simulated labor

---

C-SECTIONS

A Caesarean section—or C-section—is a surgical procedure performed to deliver a baby through the abdomen in situations when it is impossible or unadvisable to deliver the baby through the vagina. Sometimes scheduled in advance, but also done under emergency conditions, C-sections should always be a heavily weighted decision, as vaginal birth is the preferred method of delivery if possible due to higher risk for the mother during a C-section. In the United States, 32 percent of all births are delivered by C-section. Compare that number to 15 percent in the Netherlands and 25 percent in England, Wales, and Canada, and it's clear that the United States has a higher rate than other countries.[28] Our high rates may be due to factors ranging from new technology that provides increased monitoring, causing worry, to doctor's fear of lawsuits as well as to women's desire to control their delivery date.[29]

and all the pains of childbirth for themselves. Sign him up! You won't be attached to a simulator because you will be experiencing the real deal, but don't worry: There are myriad methods both natural and medical that can help you through labor and delivery. If you want, you can to draw on birthing methods, take advantage of the epidural or other forms of anesthesia, or use a combination of natural and medical to help you through the pain and on to the fun part: where you become a mom.

After giving birth, you may feel sore and swollen, but that should clear up after a few weeks. If you tore or needed to have an episiotomy—a procedure done to make more room for the baby's head during which a small cut is made to the skin called the perineum that is between the vagina and the anus—you may be contending with stiches. Peeing can burn like crazy, so many women use a squirt bottle to spray water on their vulva and vaginal opening to reduce that burning sensation. You will bleed for 2 to 6 weeks, but the volume of blood will slow down over time. For this bleeding, you should use pads and not insert anything into your vagina while you heal. So break out those granny panties and your thickest overnight pads, and try wearing loose clothing for comfort. Some women find sitting on an ice pack or a hemorrhoid ring or doughnut cushion is helpful to take some pressure of that area.

With all that your vulva and vagina have gone through, you will need time to heal. Usually your doctor will give you the green light for sex 4 to 6 weeks after giving birth. That timeframe usually is enough for you to have stopped bleeding, your cervix to have closed, and any healing that your perineum needs

BABY BLUES

Having a baby can open up the floodgates to emotion—happiness, joy, worry, fear, love, and, perhaps most unexpected reaction: depression. Within the first 2 to 3 days after delivery, the "baby blues" can set in, resulting in mood swings, crying spells, anxiety, and difficulty sleeping while your hormones even out. These fluctuations in hormones and your emotions normally last a few weeks, but some new moms suffer from a more severe, long-lasting form of emotional imbalance: postpartum depression or, even more seriously, postpartum psychosis. Talk to your doctor about these issues, because your body is not the only part of you that is impacted by giving birth—your mental health is just important as your physical, and starting treatment early is key in these situations.[31]

to have taken place. But you know your body and will be able to figure out what feels right for you. Once you are ready to have sex again, you should have a conversation with your health-care provider about birth control. You can determine what type is right for you and when you should start it. Unless you are hoping for another baby right away! *Note:* That the old wives' tale of not being able to get pregnant if you are breastfeeding your baby is not true!

Your libido may have taken a hit from the hormonal roller coaster you have been on, not to mention the fact that you may be super tired from lack of sleep—those late-night feedings can take their toll—and may generally not feel like yourself yet. The key things to keep in mind are to take it slow, use lots of lube because your vaginal walls may be a bit dry, and be prepared for sex to feel a little different. Your tissues and muscles have been stretched out pretty far and will not be back to their usual selves for a little while. Most women and their partners report that they don't feel a difference pre- and postpregnancy to the size and tightness of the vagina.[30] Just another old wives' tale! We should not be listening to all of these old wives!

Not stressing, doing some Kegel exercises, and keeping the lines of communication open with your partner can go a long way to finding your way back to satisfying sex postpregnancy.

Now that your options are laid out in front of you and you have the facts, we hope you will be able to have more productive and open conversations about both pregnancy as well as preventing pregnancy. Know that you have the freedom to choose, with the help of your doctor, what is best for you when it comes to pregnancy prevention and safer sex.

SEXUALITY 101: WHAT'S SEX AND WHAT'S SEXY?

LET'S TALK ABOUT SEX. It has probably come to your attention that the word *sex* is most commonly used in two ways: either as "Do you want to have sex?" or next to a little blank line on a medical form. One usage can inspire anything from feeling awkward to excited, and the other is simply sterile and factual, but surprise, surprise: Sex is way bigger than that. We're going to clear up some of the terminology around sex and sexuality so that you will feel comfortable using the terms as well as understand what they mean when you hear them from a partner or friend, online, or in your favorite magazine.

SEX AND GENDER IDENTITY

Facebook now offers a choice of 51 different gender options[1] to their users, and the general population's understanding and awareness of the language we use to discuss gender and sex is continuing to expand. So before we run headlong toward to the lusty, heavy-breathing definition of sex, it's worth taking a moment to address the other half of that definition and the word it so frequently gets confused with: *gender*.

SEX

The word *sex* in this case refers to biology in terms of chromosomes (most commonly XX for female or XY for male), hormones, gonads (either ovaries or testicles), reproductive units (sperm or eggs), and internal and external anatomy. While we often conceive of sex in terms of the two categories—male or female—this binary system is really inadequate for comprehensively describing the sex characteristics of our diverse population. For example, intersex individuals are born with a combination of male and female sex characteristics, and there are a multitude of chromosomal and hormonal conditions that impact development of sex characteristics.

GENDER

Gender is a term that doesn't consider your biology but describes your sense of self primarily in terms of masculine, feminine, neither, or both. Chances are, if there were pink balloons at your baby shower and—whether you prefer to wear dresses and makeup or pantsuits and a pixie cut—you have grown into someone who feels comfortable calling yourself a woman and confidently pushing open the bathroom door with the little stick figure in a dress on it, you haven't given much thought to your own gender identity. But for many, correlating male/ female sex to man/woman gender identity just doesn't do justice to their experience or who they are inside. Expanding gender terms past the binary man/woman is becoming more and more accepted and celebrated as awareness increases.

Beginning below is a short and nonexhaustive list of some of the most common gender terms that you might come across. As you read these terms and as you encounter people out in the world who use them, keep in mind that gender is a sensitive issue for many people. Remember: It's important that you let others tell you about their gender in their own time, if at all, and that you are respectful of the pronouns they use to describe themselves. This is not about being "politically correct"—it's about being a decent person who cares about the comfort and safety of those around them.

Cisgender

Frequently shortened to "cis," this is a term for people who have the gender identity that is commonly associated with their biological sex. A person who is assigned male at birth who grows up to live and identify as a man is a cis male or cis man, and a person who is assigned female at birth who grows up to live and identify as a woman is a cis female or cis woman.

Transgender

This term encompasses all individuals who have gender identities that are not associated traditionally with the sex they were assigned at birth. This includes someone who identifies as a trans man, meaning he was assigned female at birth and lives as a man—also referred to as female to male/FTM. In the same way, a trans woman is someone who was assigned male at birth and lives as a woman—also referred to as male to female/MTF.

Gender Nonconforming

People who identify as gender nonconforming look and behave in ways that do not fit into our societal expectations of gender. Similarly, persons who identify as gender fluid have a gender presentation and identity not limited by gender categories: One day they may feel more like a man and wish to wear a suit, and the next they may feel more like a woman and put on their favorite skirt and heels. Other individuals identify as gender queer, gender nonbinary, gender questioning, transfeminine, or transmasculine. Although each of these terms has its own history and importance to the individual—even the specific spelling of these words holds significance to some—they all exist under the umbrella of terms that people choose to represent themselves outside of the traditional male/female–man/ woman binary. These individuals will often use the pronouns *they/them* or other terms that they are comfortable with.

Agender

Agender individuals—who often also use the terms *genderless* or *gender neutral*—do not identify as any gender at all.

GENDER IN THIS BOOK

This book is primarily speaking directly to cisgendered women—people who were born female and live comfortably as women in their adult lives—but there is plenty here that can speak to you if you happen to be a trans man who gets a period or a trans woman who is impacted by the social issues that we cover. We aim to be inclusive and want everyone to feel welcome at Vagina University!

They/them pronouns often accompany this identity.

As we said on page 121, this list doesn't come close to covering the many different gender identities, terms, and expressions that people choose, so we encourage you to continue being open to exploring and learning about this area—even if it's only to understand all of the options available on Facebook.[2] You have your gender, so you be you and let others do the same.

Now, on to the sexy aspects of the word "sex" . . .

SEXUALITY AND SEXUAL ORIENTATION

Sexuality is an important aspect of how you see yourself and how you physically relate to other people—it's how you do you as a sexual being. Because everyone's upbringings, personalities, and experiences cover an enormous variety and range, sexuality is very individual. How you feel, think, and express yourself sexually are all part of your sexuality. How you take care of your sexual and reproductive health is part of sexuality. Sensuality and intimacy are part of your sexuality. And while, as we said, your gender identity and sex are not your sexuality, they influence your sexuality because they are a part of you. How you feel about your body and how you want to interact with others is part of sexuality, and this is biologically, socially, and culturally informed as well. With so many influences, it is no wonder that people express their sexuality in so many different ways.

With whom you interact sexually is usually a part of sexual orientation, which relates to how you define yourself and the attraction you feel (emotional and physical) to others. There is a lot of fluidity to sexual orientation, but there are three broad categories:

QUEER

The term *queer* has a complicated history. According to the *Oxford English Dictionary*, the word—which dates back to the 16th century as a synonym for "strange or odd"—appeared in the late 19th century as an aggressively derogatory term for homosexual people. By the 1980s, however, gay people took the word back, deliberately using it in a neutral way in place of "homosexual" and shouting it proudly in the popular rallying cry: "We're here, we're queer, get used to it!" Queer is now a commonly accepted word to connote not only homosexuality but any sexual or gender identity not in line with heterosexuality, although the derogatory usage still persists alongside the neutral.

- Heterosexual/straight: Opposite sex attraction
- Homosexual/gay/lesbian: Same sex attraction
- Bisexual/bi: Either sex attraction

Having said that, even these categories have their limitations. There are people who identify as asexual, meaning they are not interested in sexual relationships, and pansexual, which means that sex and gender are not factors in whom they are attracted to sexually. People of all genders can express their sexual orientation in the broad categories listed above or in other ways as well.

Most people become aware of their sexual orientation around puberty—but for some, it happens earlier and for others, later. Also, you can feel physically attracted to, or fantasize about, someone of the opposite sex or about both sexes without necessarily being homosexual or bisexual. Sexual orientation, according to most experts, is not a choice and cannot be changed. Bottom line, no one else can tell you what your orientation is—it's as personal as your fingerprint.[3, 4]

DATING ONLINE, AKA DATING

The term *dating* has become almost synonymous with "online dating" these days, and in a few swipes you can set up a date online just as easily as you can order paper towels. While some people give both activities about the same amount of thought and consideration—swiping through profile after profile in line at the grocery story or during their bathroom break—you and the rest of the 40 percent of the population who uses online dating[5] have so many options there, it's worth doing your homework to find the right site or app for what you are looking for in a match. Just looking for sex? There's an app for that. Searching for a person of your same faith? There is an app for that, too! Each site has its own algorithm, personality, perks, and drawbacks, so choose with care and remember: You can always message first, you have carte blanche to end any interaction you don't want to be in, and you are free to report any unsolicited dick-pics or other inappropriate messages.

With this new dating culture, there is a whole new set of complications and pleasures ranging from the anguish of deciding whether you want to pay to join a certain site to the joy of chatting with someone online to make a connection before you meet them IRL—building up anticipation for that first meeting. But there are also dangers inherent in meeting up with someone you met online, and while online dating is a great way to meet someone, taking some precautions to protect your privacy, until you get to know someone better, is probably a good idea.

We don't want to go off on a whole "stranger danger" riff, but we probably don't have to tell you that the first time you meet someone you have matched with online should be in a public place, right? It also can't hurt to let a friend know where you are going and who you are meeting. We're not trying to make you paranoid, but some commonsense approaches (don't get into a car with someone you don't know; texting and wink emojis don't count as "knowing"; don't share too many personal details at

SEXTING

Texting and chatting online can be a fun and flirty way to keep things heated up between you and your partner, whether you are miles away or in the same town or city. Sexting can free you to be a little more explicit than you might be in person and give you an opportunity to express yourself in ways that might leave you tongue-tied when you are face-to-face. The trick is to keep it fun and light and not to get too hard core until you know him well enough to be able to communicate on a superintimate level. Emojis can speak volumes if you don't want to put your sexy thoughts into actual words. Yes, he's probably going to ask for "noodz," but if you don't want to send them, don't. Those pics you send, that may seem fun and harmless in the moment, may come back to haunt you because texts, snaps, and anything you put out into the universe doesn't always disappear the way you may want it to—mutual trust is important here. If you want to send images, you can always send a superhot photo that doesn't include identifying characteristics or your face to keep a little mystery and protect your images for the future. So have fun, be sexy, be sexty!

first) can keep you safe. If you are swiping or selecting, take care with what and with whom you share.

One useful tip is to restrict communication to the app or site you connected through before you meet. If a potential match asks you for your number or your personal e-mail, just politely say you want to keep chatting the way you started and gauge their reaction. Do they act totally cool and understand, or do they freak out? This can help you figure out the intentions and attitude of the person on the other end of the chat. Also, it never hurts to do a quick social media search before you meet up with anyone just in case you can quickly find out that they are planning on cheating on their girlfriend with you—relationship status: busted—or if they are the type of guy who uses more #hashtags than actual words! Or you might just find that they have a cute pup named Rocket or something adorable like that— also valuable intel!

Additional information on safe use of the Internet can be found at Stop. Think. Connect. (www.stopthinkconnect.org).

PILLOW TALK

One of the times where good communication and the ability to have an open and frank discussion is very important is the first time you have sex with someone. In fact, consent is the most important aspect of communication during sex, and it's essential to be sure you are always getting and giving clear and enthusiastic consent from your partner whether you have been together for years or this is your first time together. Remember, unconscious or extremely drunk people cannot give consent, and even if you've already given consent, you should feel free to say no to any activity or behavior that makes you feel uncomfortable, unsafe, or that you don't want to engage in for any reason—or no reason at all. A yes only remains yes until someone says no.

Another conversation that has to happen before that first time is the safer sex talk. Using a condom, although not foolproof, is the best protection you have against a sexually transmitted infection or sexually transmitted disease (STI or STD), not to mention pregnancy. It can feel awkward to bring up the subject, but a simple "Do you have protection?" can get the issue out in the open. You can put yourself in the responsibility driver's seat and have condoms handy just in case, too—safer sex is a team effort. Honestly, if you are too embarrassed to bring up the topic of his wearing a condom, it's time to ask yourself if you are really ready to have his penis in your vagina. Yes, that spontaneous sex in the restroom of the bar may be exciting and fun, but you don't want those moments of pleasure to come back to haunt you later with a horrible itch or worse. His refusing to use a condom, especially the first time you have sex with him, should be a deal breaker. As mentioned previously, condoms come in many styles and designs that can enhance your sexual experience. Rather than treating putting on the condom as an unwelcome break in the action, make it part of your sex play. You can put it on him . . . slowly. You can put it on him with your mouth. Or be bold and use fun colors or glow-in-the-dark ones. Unless you are in a monogamous relationship and you have both been tested for STDs/STIs, a condom *should* come between you![6]

If there is a theme that runs through a lot of discussions about sex, it's that communication plays a very important role. Talking openly with your partner about how you like to be touched and where you want to be touched can make your sexual experience all the more fulfilling and pleasurable. Now, we're not talking about rattling off a "do this, don't do that" litany of demands every time you are in bed—unless, of course, you are playing at the provocative and powerful boss ordering around the new hire on the job. Open, honest, communication in and out of bed is respectful and involves nearly as much listening as it does talking. So it's not just about you asking for what you want, it's hearing what your partner wants, too. Talking dirty can be part of sexy play, and it doesn't have to be super-scripted or particularly eloquent. Saying "I like that!" or a simple "Harder!" may be as dirty and explicit as you want to get. Whisper if you want to, compliment your partner on what they are doing, and say how good it makes you feel. Heck, even a heartfelt moan can be just as powerful as talking dirty and turn your partner on. It can affect you, too! Expressing your pleasure can be the ultimate feedback loop in feeling sexy and letting yourself get caught up in the moment.

HAVING SEX

Sex isn't only sexual intercourse. Sex is really any behavior that you engage in with yourself or another (or multiple others) that is sexual for you. Sex can involve kissing/making out, stimulating breasts or nipples, penis in vagina, fingers in vagina, penis in mouth, penis in anus, mouth on vulva/clitoris, sex toys in vagina or anus, and any combination of all of the above. Really, as long as it is consensual, then you and your partner get to decide what it is for you and your partner. Because this is Vagina U, we'll talk primarily about sex as it pertains to those who have vaginas. Without further ado, here's the lowdown on getting down.

MASTURBATION

Although a lot of people think that masturbation is primarily for bros, it's absolutely for women, too. Women do it for pleasure, stress relief, getting in touch with their bodies, and, of course, having orgasms (duh). Solo self-pleasuring can be an excellent way to better understand your body and what feels good, and you can then use this knowledge to communicate to your partner your favorite ways to be touched and what works to get you off when you are together.

Although many people use masturbation as their form of a personal quickie or lube job just to get off and satisfied, masturbation doesn't have to be a no-frills event. You can really make a self-sex session a sensual and pleasurable experience by treating yourself to self-massage, sparking up some candlelight, using some warming lube, and relaxing in the position of your choice. Many women use their fingers to stimulate their clitoris and labia and focus on external stimulation, while others use vibrators, dildos, or fingers for both external and internal stimulation. Vibrators come in all shapes and sizes: some for clitoral stimulation, some for penetration, and some for both. Some are curved to reach that elusive G-spot. To get the most out of masturbation, and to stay out of a self-satisfaction rut, you can switch things up—hey, you might discover that vaginal stimulation brings you a different kind of pleasure or that only concentrating on your clitoris makes you superhappy. If you always use your go-to vibrator, save on those batteries and try using your fingers, or if you've always let your fingers do the work, then maybe try a vibrator or other sex toy to explore what feels good. If you only do it lying down, try sitting up or experimenting with another position that feels comfortable. How about leaving the bed behind and take a bath or shower—that handheld showerhead may do more than you think!

But while you are experiencing these new sensations and feelings, remember that there is one thing that you shouldn't have to feel during masturbation: shame. In the 1700s, a pamphlet was circulated referring to masturbation as "heinous sin of self pollution"[7]—and while some women look at that and scoff, "Well, no one believes that now, that was a long time ago . . ." others still allow these puritanical and sex-negative views to make them feel dirty and base every time they touch their bodies. But self-love is all about love—your body is yours,

---

REPLACE PAIN WITH PLEASURE

Masturbation during your period can help with cramps. When you O, your brain releases dopamine, oxytocin, and endorphins that act as a natural pain reliever. And it can also help you sleep![8] So next time you are all cramped up and huddled in front of Netflix, turn off your show and turn yourself on!

and only you decide who else gets to touch you and how you touch yourself. Shame-free self-love for everyone!

SEXUAL INTERCOURSE

Penetrative, vaginal sex is when the penis is inserted into the vagina, thrusts in and out to create friction, typically leading to orgasm—ideally for both parties involved—and the ejaculation of semen into the vagina. When you have vaginal sex, you can protect yourself from sexually transmitted diseases and unintended pregnancy by using a condom, and prevent pregnancy through using one of the other forms of birth control (see Chapter 3).

The whole process sounds pretty simple, but what happens to your vagina and surrounding areas during sex is anything but! If a man is aroused, his erect and engorged penis is a pretty obvious indication that he's ready for some action, but for a woman, the signs are more subtle and interior. Bloodflow increases in the vulva, and the vagina begins to secrete fluids, aka "getting wet." Your clitoris will also gain increased bloodflow and will actually expand and stiffen in the same way a penis gets hard. From either side of the vaginal opening, the Bartholin's glands get in on the action and release a bit of slippery mucus to aid in your self-lube. The cervix softens, and if it is reached by extra-deep thrusting or probed by a sex toy, it can get some pleasure going also!

Some women do not orgasm during vaginal sex—even if they are able to orgasm during masturbation—likely due to the clitoris not getting enough stimulation. If that's happening to you, it's time to change positions or give more attention to your little love button before intercourse.

When you orgasm, the pelvic floor and vagina have muscle contractions that can feel sexy for both you and your partner. Sometimes a woman can have some fluid come out of her urethra during orgasm, which can come as a bit of a surprise, but it is not urine, so don't worry if this happens to you. About 10 percent of women ejaculate during sex, and you can actually learn how to squirt or gush during sex if that appeals to you. It can take some practice, but we think you might enjoy this homework: The key is getting in touch with your G-spot, and close to that is the Skene gland, which is the source of female ejaculate. If you have ever felt the urge to pee when you are about to orgasm, you may have naturally clenched up, but that feeling is triggered by ejaculate coming from the Skene gland—and if you let go, you may come with fluid. Before you have sex, make sure you pee beforehand so you don't have to worry about urination issues. Having vaginal sex from behind gives you a better chance of his penis hitting the G-spot, but you can get there yourself by hooking a finger up behind the pubic bone with the cup of your hand on your clitoris

---

LADY BONERS

The clitoris and the penis have something in common other than that they are key players in sexual activity. They are similar glands that share a common initial state in the embryo. They both have erectile tissue, so you really can get a little lady boner when you are aroused!

to keep stimulation going there. For gushing or squirting to happen, you will need to be super aroused and to apply a fair amount of pressure to the G-spot and in turn the Skene gland. If squirting doesn't happen for you, NBD. But keep practicing, because you never know when you can hit the jackpot!

ANAL SEX

Your "back door" can be a source of pleasure, but some women are hesitant to engage in anal sex or anal sex play. As with all aspects of sexual activity, there is no pressure on where you get your pleasure, so if anal is something you want to try, go for it. If the thought makes you uncomfortable, then maybe it's not for you. Here are some ideas on how to keep butt play safe and fun. If anal sex brings to mind being dirty, messy, or painful, it doesn't have to be that way. Washing up beforehand can take away some of the concern for cleanliness, and as to discomfort and if you are concerned about the poop factor, you can make yourself go to the bathroom before getting into butt action and have a bowel movement so that it's all clear for play—or try using a water-based enema.[9] To avoid risk of infection, don't put anything into your anus and then put it into your vagina. This goes for toys, fingers, and penises. Use a condom to protect yourself from bacterial infection or STDs/STIs.[10]

There are other things you can do to minimize the pain and maximize your pleasure as well. The trick is to take it slowly and use lots and lots of lube, preferably silicone based. A little self-exploration in the shower where you can be relaxed and warm can give you ideas about what feels good and what doesn't. Inserting a lubed finger into your own anus and contracting the sphincter muscles can help you to discover what you may like if you engage in anal play with a partner using a penis or sex toy. Because the skin around the anus doesn't have any natural lubrication, is sensitive, and can tear, it is very important to go slowly. Be sure you are fully aroused and fully lubed before inserting anything into your anus, and if it is painful, slow down, back off a little, and did we mention that it helps to breathe? Yep, breathing steadily can keep those muscles from tensing up and blocking entry. During anal penetration or play, stimulation of your clitoris or vagina can get you more bang for your buck, and be sure to communicate with your partner about what feels good and what doesn't. Over time, anal sex can loosen the sphincter muscles, so those trusty Kegels can keep the area toned and prevent any leakage. Because of the lack of lubrication and the sensitive tissues back there, you may see some bleeding after anal sex; a small amount is pretty normal. If you are bleeding excessively or have discharge, then please check in with your doctor.[11]

ORAL SEX

Mouth on labia and clitoris can lead to fabulous orgasms as long as the stimulation isn't too much, too fast or too little, too slow—you get the idea—what feels good to you is what feels good to you. It's normal to feel a little self-conscious when your significant other is "going down" on your lady parts. It is where you pee, after all, and everyone has her own personal scent, discharge, and appearance. It can make you feel less self-conscious if you pee beforehand and then do a little extra cleanup in aisle V. If you use a feminine wipe to freshen up, be sure it is one that is fragrance-free, alcohol-free, and glycerin-free, because it's best not to use anything with additives that can potentially cause irritation.

Interestingly, what you eat may influence your scent down there. Foods that can throw off your naturally acidic pH can affect the taste and smell of your vagina—coffee, alcohol, asparagus, onions, and garlic can all influence the scent of a woman. The same goes for men: Some scientists speculate that drinking lots of water and eating a diet rich in fruits and veggies can improve the taste of his ejaculate.[12]

A traditional position for receiving oral sex is you lying back with your partner's mouth on your muff, but you can also try sitting on a counter with your partner in front of you, keeling over your partner's mouth, or—for added degree of difficulty and as a way to ratchet up the pleasure for both of you—try the 69 position, where you perform oral sex on your partner while they simultaneously perform it on you. This can be done lying on top of each other or facing each other side by side. To protect against sexually transmitted diseases or infection, you can use a dental dam or condom.

LIKE A VIRGIN . . .

The definition of virginity isn't as clear-cut as you might think. Virginity is most commonly defined as never having had sexual intercourse, and many people think of losing your virginity as having vaginal penetrative intercourse—specifically, penis-in-vagina sex. But are you are virgin if you have had oral or anal sex? If you are not heterosexual and engage in sexual activity that does not involve vaginal sex, are you still a virgin? Ultimately, how you define being a virgin largely depends on your sexuality, background, and culture.

There is a common misconception that if a woman loses or tears the stretchy tissue near the opening of the vagina, called the hymen, she is no longer a virgin, or "intact." Her "cherry" has been popped. The hymen, however, can be torn through activities like sports, horseback riding, and using tampons, so a torn hymen does not make you not-a-virgin. It might mean that you just really like doing the splits in gymnastics. On the other hand, some women never tear their hymens at all as, contrary to popular belief, the hymen doesn't actually cover the vaginal opening and can accommodate fingers, tampons, and, yes, a penis. Women's bodies don't come fitted with virginity detectors or freshness seals, and yet the hymen test has been used as a measure of virginity for eons. Even today, many people don't understand this aspect of female anatomy.[13]

The first time you have vaginal sex—penis in vagina—or a finger is inserted into the vagina, it may hurt, and there may be some bleeding. The pain and bleeding can be due to tearing of the hymen or the result of tense muscles, not enough preparation or lubrication, or inexperience. Not everyone will bleed or feel pain the first time they have vaginal intercourse. Tell that to the people in the olden days who would check the sheets of newlyweds for spots of blood to confirm that the bride was a virgin...

Some cultures still place a great deal of importance on virginity, even going so far as to conduct "virginity tests" on girls for proof of virginity before marriage. And yes, those tests often entail the inspection of the hymen—the test that, as we just explained, doesn't prove anything. Religious, social, and family background play a lot into whether or not you think being a virgin or losing your virginity is important, but no matter your views, it's a moment that most women don't take lightly and that they remember for their entire lives. We hope that as more information and knowledge about sex spreads, more women remember that first time as fun, pleasurable, and free from shame—even if the act itself is still a bit fumbly and awkward.

LIKE A VIRGIN . . . AGAIN?

So you've had sex, but because of a lack of partner, lack of desire, or other extenuating circumstances, you have found yourself celibate for a long time. In your pseudo-virginal state, what happens when you have sex again? While you can't really ever be a virgin again, and although your vagina doesn't really get "tighter" after not having sex for a while,[14] having sex after a dry spell can feel as exciting and uncomfortable as the first time. Following a period where you have not engaged in sexual activity, your muscles will be unaccustomed to having sex, so you may be a little sore afterward.[15] If you are feeling physically uncomfortable, more lube, more foreplay, and more communication can help the situation. If your muscles shut down barring any entry, you may be suffering from vaginismus (see pages 150–151).

If you go through a dry spell, a great way to keep yourself prepped for when you are ready to hit the sheets again is to masturbate. Doing so will give you the benefits of orgasmic relief— all those feel-good hormones are good for you—and keep your vagina primed for when you are ready for sex with a partner. A little "me time" can get your well primed for "we time."

SEXUAL POSITIONS

The legendary *Kama Sutra* has hundreds of sex positions that require various levels of flexibility (and a dose of creativity) to achieve sexual satisfaction. A read through a hard copy of the book can inspire you to Cirque du Soleil–level heights, but you can also go high tech with apps for your phone or tablet that show illustrations and instruction for numerous sexual positions. Despite the multitude of ways you can insert tab A into slot B, before you think you have to twist yourself into a pretzel to get happy, you don't. We can't get into all the positions—even if we wanted to—so following are some tried and true positions[16] (and a couple of variations) that you are likely familiar with, but you never know . . .

So get creative and find pleasure with these positions with the partner of your choice. Feel free to play and find what works best for you and your partner. A word of advice: Go slow

---

SEXY FUN FOR EVERYONE

In most of the descriptions in this chapter, we are referring to male to female, penis-in-vagina–style sex, but these positions could be just as useful for two ladies using a strap-on or—with some modification—a handheld dildo.

---

and talk it through when you are trying a new position for having sex. Unexpected angles and placement of body parts can cause pain and possibly small tears in your vag. Ouch!

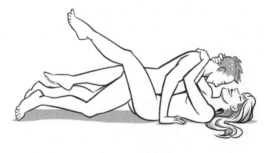

MISSIONARY

With your partner on top, you can look into one another's eyes and feel that smooth skin-to-skin contact you both crave, increasing your level of intimacy. The friction of him thrusting inside of you gives you vaginal stimulation as well as some clitoral stimulation. While this is the most vanilla of all positions, you can spice it up by lifting your legs over his shoulders or bringing them up to wrap around his waist. Or you can reverse it, with you lying on top of him. You will have more control over the motion if you are on top.

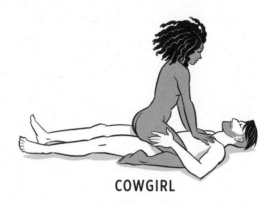

COWGIRL

Speaking of girl on top, with the cowgirl position you are on top, kneeling over him, and you have more control on the depth of penetration as well as how fast and hard you thrust. He also has clear access to your clitoris to add to your pleasure. A variation on this one is reverse cowgirl, where you face away from him. He then has access to your butt and can add some anal stimulation to the play.

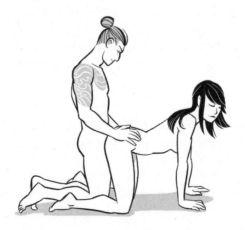

DOGGY STYLE

If it's unrestricted butt access you are after, doggy style is your position! With you on hands and knees and him penetrating your vagina from behind, he can get very deep, which can be very pleasurable as long as he takes his time with thrusting so it doesn't cause pain. We're talking long and strong here, not jackhammer. You can do a version of doggy style by lying side by side in spoon position (he is the big spoon) and he enters you from behind. This is a great modification for sex while pregnant!

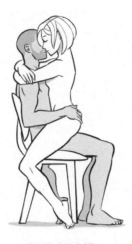

THE CHAIR

In another position that gives you plenty of control, "the chair" has your partner sitting on the bed, his back supported by pillows, or in a literal chair and you sitting on his lap facing him. You are largely in charge with how actively you are thrusting, and this position will give you some deep, toe-curling penetration. A variation on this one would be you sitting on the edge of the bed with your butt toward the edge of the bed and your legs open and over the edge with him standing between them. Because he is standing in front of you, it's also pretty easy for him to reach your clitoris for extra stimulation from this position.

THE BIG "O" . . . WHEN SEX FEELS GOOD

Merriam-Webster's dictionary defines *orgasm* as: intense or paroxysmal excitement, especially: the rapid pleasurable release of neuromuscular tensions at the height of sexual arousal that is usually accompanied by the ejaculation of semen in the male and by vaginal contractions in the female.

When they put it that way, it sounds like a lot of fun, right? What this definition doesn't mention is that, whether solo or with a partner, orgasms feel ahhhh . . . some! So what's happening in your genitals to get you to this place of bliss? As you get aroused, the bloodflow to your vagina and clitoris increases, and fluid is secreted in the walls of your vagina helping out with lubrication (also known as getting "wet"). You may also blush, flush, or start to get a little sweaty. As you continue to become more excited, your heart rate increases, your breathing becomes heavier, your nipples become erect, and a lot of muscle pressure builds up in your pelvic area and your vagina. When, because of continued stimulation, that muscle pressure releases, you are riding the wave of the Big O. Contractions that are really close together contribute to a more intense orgasm, and contractions that are less frequent lead to a less intense but also pleasurable orgasm.

The source of orgasm can be from stimulation of the clitoris or the vagina or a combination of both. If, when you are having sex, you don't reach orgasm, it is most likely because you are not getting enough stimulation of your clitoris. Getting more attention to your pleasure button can be achieved by a woman-on-top position. Something else that can get in the way is thinking too much about what is happening, if it is happening, and when it is going to happen. How to fix this? You need to get out of your head and back into bed. It's a weird phenomenon, but relaxing will actually allow your muscles to build enough pressure to get to that oh-so-great release.[17] In other words, relax and go with the flow to achieve the Big O.

If you do not get to orgasm from vaginal sex, then you are not alone: More than 50 percent of women do not achieve orgasm by penis-in-vagina sex. In the "it's not fair" department, dudes will more reliably get to orgasm during sex—yes, they have us beat on this and with the gender pay gap. Reasons for the "no O" can range from not enough time fooling around before sex to not getting enough clit attention to having your mind on that work presentation instead of your pleasure zones. Also, orgasms can sometimes be elusive as well as not feel the same from one sexual experience to another. You don't have to be shouting the roof off to be having a satisfying orgasm . . . you don't even have to shout at all!

Open communication and lots of foreplay can help you get to O town. Sometimes, shifting your focus to the pleasure you are feeling, instead of waiting for the O to happen, can help you relax and—surprise!—have that fireworks-on-the-Fourth-of-July orgasm. And if you want to find another source of pleasure, don't forget your breasts. Did you know there is such a thing as a nipple-gasm? Some women can achieve orgasm through stimulation—touching, licking, sucking—of their nipples and breasts.[18] Another fun way to play to add to your repertoire in the boudoir.

Your muscles are not the only part of you put into action through orgasm. A hormone called oxytocin, released when you climax, not only allows for some serious contractions in your

THE ORGASM GAP

According to the *Archives of Sexual Behavior,* a February 2017 study reported this demographic data of those groups who "usually-always orgasmed" when sexually intimate:

DEMOGRAPHIC GROUP	FREQUENCY OF ORGASM
Heterosexual men	95 percent
Gay men	89 percent
Bisexual men	88 percent
Lesbian women	86 percent
Bisexual women	66 percent
Heterosexual women	65 percent

The heterosexual women who more often experienced orgasm were more likely to be in a satisfying relationship, experienced oral sex, engaged in deep kissing and fantasies, and were able to ask for what they wanted in bed.[20]

If you are a heterosexual woman, the statistics don't seem to be in your favor, but don't give up! You can certainly have a lot of fun trying to beat the odds.

uterus but is responsible for that postsex want-to-cuddle feeling. Oxytocin is often known as the love hormone or the bonding hormone. In addition to the oxytocin, your brain releases endorphins that are responsible for feeling good—they are the same hormones that are responsible for the legendary "runner's high." Those endorphins are also the reason why you may not experience pain from a neck nibble or scratches on your back in the throes of passion but find that you are sore afterward. Those feel-good hormones serve as pain blockers, too. Another part of the brain, the amygdala (responsible for anxiety and fear), basically shuts down when you have an orgasm, which is why it seems like your brain kind of goes blank when you O.[19]

THE BIG "OH NO!" . . . WHEN SEX DOESN'T FEEL RIGHT

If you experience pain during sex, and it is not intentional, there are some simple actions you can take to keep things delightful and not uncomfortable. One of the primary and most common causes of pain or discomfort during sex is lack of lubrication. When your vag is making like the Sahara Desert, it could be because of where you are in your cycle or the type of birth control you use. Other possible causes for dry vagina could be stress or antihistamines—they are meant to dry up the mucous membranes in your nose, but they can also have an impact on your vagina. If you feel drier than normal, you may need a little more preamble (who could say no to more foreplay?) before you get to it, and even when you do—lube to the rescue!

If you discover that you are bleeding after sex, whether or not it is a problem depends on how much bleeding and for how long you bleed. A little blood can be normal, as the tissues at the entrance to the vagina are sensitive and can be torn or damaged during enthusiastic sex. Or you might just be starting your period, so an awareness of where you are in your cycle can help determine if the blood is no big deal or something that needs medical attention. If you are bleeding a lot and are experiencing pain, you need to get medical help—like at the ER—right away.

Itching or burning could be caused by an allergic reaction to a lube, spermicide, or condom, especially if you have never used a particular brand before. You can have a reaction if you have a latex allergy, as many condom brands are made of latex. If he wasn't using any protection, then you could actually be allergic to his sperm (it's a thing!). If sperm allergy turns out to be the case, simply using a condom can prevent your having an itchy reaction. A rash or itchiness can also be caused by products he has used to clean his penis or pubes, so ask if he's using something different. A new soap or body spray for him could lead to a problem for you. Or itching may be the result of a yeast or other infection, so you'll want to have that checked out by your gyno to be sure (see pages 200–202).

Can your honey be too well hung? It is possible that your vagina and his penis are not a, well, perfect fit, but there are strategies you can take to successfully, and pleasurably, insert large tab A into a smaller slot B. Most vaginas can accommodate most penises, but sometimes you can run into a little trouble. Entry may be difficult if you are too dry, so adding more lube and more foreplay can help ease the way in. If he feels like he is getting blocked by something in your vagina, it could be that he is hitting your cervix and you are not yet ready for that level of contact: As part of the arousal process, the uterus lifts and the vagina expands; if you jump into things too fast without enough foreplay, it can feel as if there is no room for him in your V. Take a little more time, have some fun, and your body will react and become receptive. If he really is large and you are petite, try changing sexual positions so you will have more control over how deep he is going into your vagina.

WHEN MORE LUBE AND FOREPLAY AREN'T CUTTING IT

If it hurts when you are having sex, talk with your partner and see if a change of position, an addition of lube, or bit more pre-penetration play can help. But if pain happens frequently or if you have pain after sex that lasts for more than a couple of days, talk to your doctor and have the situation evaluated. In addition to these more general issues, there are a few specific disorders that you may encounter.[21]

Ovarian Cysts or Endometriosis
If you feel deep pain during sex, it is possible that you have an ovarian cyst or that it is a sign of endometriosis, a disorder that

causes the tissue that is normally inside your uterus to grow outside of your uterus. Because the tissue still responds to hormonal cues to grow and shed, it can be the source of intense pain as the tissue has nowhere to go when it breaks down and thus can lead to cysts, irritation, and scar tissue.

If you have endometriosis, you can have painful periods, pain with intercourse, and heavy bleeding. It can also lead to infertility. The cause for endometriosis hasn't been definitively determined, but it is thought that it could be due to menstrual blood flowing back into the fallopian tubes, or it could have some connection to an immune system disorder or possibly a hormonal imbalance. It can begin shortly after your first period. Ultrasound and a procedure called a laparoscopy—an outpatient procedure to view inside the abdomen—are most typically used to diagnose endometriosis.

Pain meds, hormone therapy, and occasionally surgery are the usual approaches to resolving endometriosis. If fertility has been impacted, and a woman wants to have a baby, then fertility treatments can be used to help her get pregnant.[22]

From Lena Dunham to Halsey to Padma Lakshmi,[23] celebrities have recently been opening up to the media about their struggles with endometriosis, bringing awareness for the first time to this long-misunderstood and silent condition that impacts 1 in 10 women.

Vaginismus

If your vagina feels like it is completely shutting down in response to penetration, you may be suffering from vaginismus:

a painful condition that is treatable with dedication, patience and persistence. Although the cause is unproven, many patients have a psychological component such as anxiety or sexual abuse that may be at the root of this disorder. The muscles at the entrance to the vagina clench or even spasm so that penetration is painful at best or at worst impossible. The solution is slowly stretching the muscles, often using slender dilators from your doctor made of plastic, metal, or silicone that familiarize the body with the sensation so that the muscles won't clam up when you want to get it on. Kegels can give you some relief (see pages 15–16), and Botox has been found to help. Speak with your doctor about the issue. She can guide you to the best solution for you.

MIND YOUR P WHEN YOU O

Some women pee during sex or orgasm! Usually it is the result of a weak pelvic floor—so remember to do your Kegels—but it can just be due to a full bladder. If it happens often, talk to your doctor.

Vulvodynia

Extreme burning pain in the vulva and around the entrance to the vagina can be the result of something called vulvodynia, the cause of which is a bit of a mystery, as it is not linked to a particular infection or disease. It can make sex or even trying to insert a tampon painful; it can also be uncomfortable to walk around, move, or sit down. Women have found relief through medications such as anti-inflammatories, local anesthetics, or antidepressants. Any pain that follows you around all day needs to be checked out by your doctor.

Dyspareunia

If you have dyspareunia, you will experience pain during or after having sex. The pain could be felt in your clitoris, labia, or in your vagina and has a number of causes that are relatively easy to treat. It can be due to dryness, medications you may be taking, inflammation, or even psychological trauma. A very common cause is endometriosis. Your doctor can help you determine the root cause of the pain based on your symptoms and medical history.

THINGS THAT "EVERYONE" KNOWS ABOUT SEX . . .

Oh, that "everyone" . . . spreading myths and misinformation everywhere she (or he) goes! There are many misunderstandings about sex that people will swear are true[24] but in reality, "everyone" doesn't know as much as you might think.

THE BIGGER THE BETTER

Penis size is a perennial in the world of sex myths. The mythologizing goes that more is more, until you get to those other myths about some men being "too big." Not sure you can have it both ways, but no matter what his size, you can find a way to pleasure without a problem. If he is "smaller," then you can try sex in positions that allow him to penetrate deeply, like good old missionary. If he really is big, then you may want to take charge and be able to control how deep and how fast you have sex: Try riding him like a cowgirl and you'll be able to handle his size. As mentioned on page 149, it takes some time for your vagina to expand as you become aroused, so "too big" may in reality be a result of "too soon."

FOOD FOR THOUGHT

You have probably heard that some foods are known aphrodisiacs that, should you eat them, will definitely get you in the mood. A number of foods have been given credit for inspiring those sexy feelings: raw oysters, chocolate, champagne, bananas, and watermelon. Modern science has identified components of these foods that could lead to increased arousal and better sex, like the citrulline in watermelon that increases nitric oxide in the blood and boosts circulation, or the phenylethylamine in dark chocolate that stimulates dopamine (a feel-good hormone). Can eating aphrodisiacs get you in the mood? Maybe. But by enjoying and sharing some of these delicious foods with your significant other, you may end up feeling something more than full at the end of your meal. No guarantees on the food, but an intimate meal with your partner can bring you closer together and make you both want to get busy. So enjoy these foods if you like them, but they may not get you aroused any more than anything else you can eat.

Speaking of things you put in your mouth, "everyone" knows that sperm is high in calories and full of protein, right? Actually, not so much. The only danger to swallowing sperm is if your guy has an STI, otherwise it is sterile and basically calorie-free—a normal male ejaculation contains only 5 to 25 calories per teaspoon and a minimal amount of protein.[25]

RISK-FREE PERIOD SEX

Although most people believe that you cannot get pregnant if you have sex during your period, it is definitely possible. Sperm can be tenacious. If you have vaginal sex even when you are menstruating, those little swimmers can live inside your body for 3 to 5 days. So use a condom or other protection if you are having sex, even when you are on your period, if you do not want to get pregnant. If you are icked out by having sex when you are bleeding, skip intercourse and engage in some mutual masturbation or the sex play of your choice . . . but otherwise just lay down a towel to protect your sheets and play on.

POST-SEX PEE BREAK

It's a good idea to go and pee after having sex, as it will flush out any bacteria that could have entered your urethra during sex and may save you from getting an itch or an annoying infection that you don't want to deal with.

WRAP IT UP

Condoms themselves have lots of myths surrounding their usage. First, let's be clear that a condom provides protection against pregnancy *and* sexually transmitted diseases. So what's with the myths that keep people from using them? Well, there's the perennial misconception that condoms reduce sensitivity and make sex feel less good. While it is true that a condom can cause more friction and lead to discomfort, as with lots of issues surrounding sex, lube is the answer. Also, there are a vast number of types and styles of condoms, including those that are ribbed, dotted, textured, flavored, colored, and much more (glow in the dark, anyone?). With all the choices available, you can find one that works for you and your partner. Another factor in condom avoidance is a belief that condoms can cause UTIs. Not true. These infections are caused by bacteria, tears, or irritation that result from going hard without enough lubrication. Don't let the bad intel keep you from using a rubber when you need one, and be sure to follow a "no glove, no love" policy.

FEELING SEXY—TURN-ONS (AND TURN-OFFS)

Libido, sex drive, and feeling horny are the results of a complex interplay of hormones and basically where you are mentally, physically, and emotionally. Like your sexuality, it is very individual, and everyone has his or her own natural levels of desire, but even that is not a predictable constant and can vary over time.

The basics of arousal are that the brain releases chemicals into your system that trigger physical responses—heart pounding, sweaty palms, heavy breathing—that signal that you are feeling a little naughty. But this doesn't always happen, so if you don't constantly feel like a teenager at the drive-in, it doesn't mean you are no longer attracted to your partner. Also, you may have a different level of sex drive with one partner versus another or you may have lower drive when you are going through a difficult life situation or are exhausted or are stressed from work or are having conflicts in your relationship. The key is to know yourself and understand what is standard operating sexual behavior for you. Sex once a week may be your norm, while for someone else it is once a day, and for someone else multiple times a day may be his or her usual lust level. It's another case of needing to know yourself and knowing your own version of "normal" so that you can take action if things become not normal for you. What to watch for is a change in your level of desire. If you notice a dip, to try to determine what may be putting out your fire.

DAMPENING DESIRE

There are a host of reasons that may leave you feeling blasé about banging. For guys, it's frequently all about the bloodflow, which is why drugs like Viagra work to help men get it up and get it on. For women, there's usually a bit more going on that isn't easily treatable by a pill. A lot is happening in your body and your life that fuels your lust levels, and a number of factors can derail you from getting happily busy between the sheets with your partner. Following are some of those mood killers and suggestions on how you can get your groove back![26]

Stress

The hormone that is released when we feel stressed is called cortisol, and it is a natural and necessary part of our chemical makeup, but unfortunately, when it is produced over a long period of time, it can suppress sex hormones, lowering libido. Too much stress can take a toll on relationships as well: No one wants to be around a snappish, grumpy stress case, let alone have sex with one. De-stress by having a bath, taking a breath, masturbating, kissing your partner, and kissing your stress good-bye.

Rough Patch

In a similar vein, if your relationship is going through a rough patch, sex may feel like the last thing you want to do. Working to clear up these life or emotional issues can put your libido back on track.

Hormones

Good old hormones are always at play when sex is the subject. Here, the hormones in your birth control pills could be putting the lockdown on your libido. The hormones in your combination birth control pill may be interfering with your body's producing testosterone, which is the hormone that drives desire. However, before you chuck out your pills, talk with your doctor about the possibility of taking a different form of birth control pills that might not have the same negative impact on your libido. Or you can explore your options for other types of birth control (see Chapter 3).

Medications

Some antidepressants or antianxiety medications can limit lust because they increase serotonin, and too much serotonin can reduce your ability to be aroused as well as leave you uninterested in sex. Other medications for treating mental health issues do not have this effect, so speak with the doctor who prescribed your meds to see if a different prescription can help with your depression or anxiety and not wipe out your desire. You do not have to trade in your sexual health in order to maintain your mental health. Report any troubling side effects to you doctor to explore alternatives and weigh the pros and cons of switching meds. Never stop taking a medication without checking with the prescribing doctor first. Other medications that can lower your libido include antacids, high blood pressure medications, antihistamines, and decongestants, so check with your medical professional if you notice a change in your sex drive when you are taking any of these types of meds. If the medication is short-term, then you may just have to ride out the episode of low libido. If it is a long-term medication, speak with your doctor about alternatives.

Headaches

The proverbial "not tonight, I have a headache" can feel like it's a legit excuse (who can get horny when having a headache?), but in reality sex can help with headaches, and that orgasm that releases muscle tension in your body can help your headache go away. Also, all those feel-good neurotransmitters that are released via the big O can reduce the pain of severe headaches like migraines or cluster headaches.

Alcohol

Good old alcohol can get in the way of sex, so don't overindulge if you want to have a big O. As William Shakespeare said in *Macbeth*, "it provokes the desire, but it takes away the performance."

Don't assume a desire dry spell is forever. Too much alcohol, not enough sleep, not feeling well, intimacy issues, and too much going on in your life are all likely to reduce your lust levels, but these can be temporary. If you are not feeling frisky, think about what might be getting in the way. Once you identify the problem, you have a better chance of fixing it.

WHEN HE IS HOT, AND YOU ARE NOT, OR VICE VERSA

Even in a long-term relationship, your and your partner's desire for sex can be on different levels; other times it can feel as if they are in completely different ZIP codes. The stereotype is that guys want sex anywhere, anytime. There is some truth to that in some men. But if your partner is feeling like making love and you feel like making Z's, it's important to first see if you can determine why you are not in the mood (see pages 156–159 for common reasons for lost libido) and take action. Occasionally, going with the motion and having sex even if you are not

100 percent gung ho is actually a good idea, because you may find yourself turned on and having fun. We're not talking about being coerced or guilted into having sex, because that is just not right, not healthy, and not good for you. We're talking about basically saying, "What the hell," and going for it even if you were practically half out of bed and about to get your day started or if you just wanted to roll over and sleep. Studies have shown that the more sex you have, the more sex you want, so getting busy— even if you aren't 100 percent all in—can connect you with your partner, keep those sexy juices flowing, and segue into fun.[27]

It is quite possible that you and your significant other have mismatched libidos, in which case you will need to find ways to keep both of you happy and satisfied by finding the frequency of sex that is just right for both of you. When you are feeling out of sync, maybe you can try touching each other without the goal of having sex. Explore each other's bodies with hands or tongues and find ways to give and get pleasure that aren't intercourse. Bring a little play into the bedroom and you may find yourself getting in the mood, and once you do, try something new to shake things up. Try different position, add a sex toy, or engage in fantasy or role-playing. Getting busy on the regular can keep your passion primed, and it can help if you masturbate, too!

Don't forget that touch is a powerful connector. Feel free to nuzzle your partner's neck or hold hands while you watch TV. Cuddle just for the comfort of it. Touch your partner just because. No, it's not the same as mind-blowing, superorgasmic sex, but it can, quite literally, keep you in touch and connected with your partner.

THE BRAIN IS THE SEXIEST ORGAN

Your brain engages in sex. Well, more accurately, your brain is activated by the various stimulations you receive during sex. Your clitoris, vagina, and nipples being touched, licked, or stroked lights up your brain . . . and helps ignite your arousal and climax.

SEX . . . IT'S ALL IN YOUR HEAD

Your brain is a powerful partner in sexual behavior. What you are thinking and feeling during sex can enhance or detract from the experience. Even in the midst of sex that you are enjoying, your brain is always on the go and can conjure up thoughts from "Can the neighbors hear us?" to "OMG, I didn't shave my legs!" If your brain is running down the details of your next business meeting or cataloging your physical flaws (those really probably *are* all in your head), you will be less likely to have an engaged experience with your partner. If your mind is ticking away, then try making direct eye contact. If you can hold your lover's gaze, even fleetingly, then you are less likely to continue being preoccupied with your work crisis du jour. Another way to bring yourself back to the moment is to focus on touch and feeling. Run your fingers through your partner's hair or nibble an earlobe: Getting your brain focused on sensory stimulation can ground you and bring you back to the moment.

A little positive self-talk can also get you ready for sex as well as keep you in the moment. Telling yourself that you are looking forward to sex will actually set your brain working in the right direction. Focusing on the pleasure you are feeling during sex, rather than either focusing on the end result or on the things that are getting in your way of pleasure, will reinforce the pleasure for you. You can also visualize yourself in postcoital bliss; holding that image in your mind can get you to that reality. Another way to engage your brain to achieve better sex is to use music, especially music that evokes memories of connection with your partner or of previous enjoyable sexual encounters. Barry White, Barry Gibb, Barry Manilow, no judgment: Whatever works for you!

FANTASIES

They sky is the limit in terms of fantasy scenarios when you are alone. You can imagine yourself in any situation or with any partner or partners. Want to imagine you are a damsel in distress being saved by the strong knight, even though you are a feminist in real life? Go for it. Imagining something that turns you on doesn't mean you have to want that action in your real life to be fulfilled—it's just for fun! Fantasy can also come into play when you are with your significant other, but sometimes those thoughts can be jarring. Sometimes, in the middle of the action, that celeb crush might pop into your mind, and although you may feel a little guilty, rest assured it is normal. Just redirect those thoughts to your real-life, in-the-flesh, in-the-bed partner and save those celeb crush fantasies for when you are solo.

When you are with your partner, probably the most difficult aspects of fantasies are admitting you have them and/or asking your partner to share them. Sharing your sexual fantasies with your partner can be blush inducing, but it can also lead to deeper intimacy—even if you never get around to acting out the fantasy. Talking about your fantasies may lead to the two of you finding new ways to please each other and opening up the lines of communication, a win-win all around.

Here are a few common fantasies to get you started.[28]

- Play boss and employee.
- Watch each other masturbate.
- Have sex outside.
- Have sex somewhere where you might get caught.
- Have sex with a "stranger" (use wigs, clothes, or props to transform your significant other into a significant "unknown").
- Play with domination/submission.

It's all up to you and your imagination.

ROLE-PLAYING

Role-playing is a common way for couples to change things up in the bedroom (or the kitchen table or the bathroom or the hallway or the car) when they act out a fantasy. Whether you only talk yourselves through the fantasy—kind of like the play-by-play of a sports announcer—or go all the way and use props and costumes, engaging in role-playing can be freeing. So tap into your hidden inner actor and let out a side of you that wants to play and put on a performance. Get him to pick you up at a bar, pretend he's the sexy handyman coming to fix the sink, or embrace that damsel-in-distress scenario and put on a princess dress—it's up to you. Get weird! It can be sexy and exciting (that's the point), but it should also be fun.

As long as you both agree to the scenario and what will happen when you act it out, go ahead and unleash the drama! Be sure to have some way of letting your partner know if things get uncomfortable or if you feel they have gone too far. It's only fun if both of you are into the role-playing and acting out the fantasy, not so much if only one partner is completely dominating the situation.

PORN

If you feel like you are lacking in the imagination department and coming up with interesting and sexy scenarios isn't your strong suit, then you can turn to porn and erotica for inspiration. There is a lot that is available to you that can suit any taste from feminist porn to hard-core. Keep in mind that your fantasies and what you enjoy watching on porn sites may not match up with your politics or even how you want to be treated in bed. Porn can get your juices flowing, but what you watch doesn't necessarily reflect how you want to personally engage in sex or be treated in bed.

Frankly, it doesn't even have to be porn: You can watch a

BROADEN YOUR SEARCH

Women can be aroused physiologically by a wide range of sexual stimuli, including naked male and female bodies, heterosexual sex, and homosexual sex. So the next time you are looking for porn to watch or looking at sexy pictures online, maybe click through some links you normally wouldn't think of and see where that takes you!

---

wide range of films and television shows for inspiration, too! You could even go old school and read an erotic novel. Try acting out a superhot sex scene from your favorite movie, TV show, or book. If traditional films or TV don't work for you, then some X-rated porn can be a source of fantasies and be used to inspire you and your partner to try something different to shake up your routine. Watching porn together can also be a way to start a conversation about something you might want to try but aren't sure how to bring up. Saying "That looks like fun!" is probably much easier than explaining and sketching out a whole scenario that you'd like to try. Porn in and of itself can serve to get you in the mood and get your juices flowing.

You may have slightly different tastes as to what you like and want to watch and what your partner likes. Give each other an opportunity to each choose a favorite and watch it together. Have some open and honest communication about what you like, or don't like, about what you watched.

Although watching porn can get you hot and heavy, it can potentially take a toll on a woman's self-image. All those perfect women, perfectly groomed, and perfectly pleasing their partners can set an unrealistic bar for flawless bodies, prolonged sex, and Oscar-worthy orgasms. Every. Single. Time. Porn can play a role in your sexual fantasies—when you are alone and when you are together—but you and your partner should always be the stars of your own sex life.

BDSM

The erotic book and movie *50 Shades of Grey* brought attention to and a shed a spotlight on sexual play involving BDSM—an acronym for bondage, domination, submission, and sadism-masochism. Of course, people have been engaging in these forms of sexual play for ages. The Marquis de Sade, from whom we get the word *sadism,* wrote a novel in 1791 that featured sex with accessories including whips and restraints. Then Leopold von Sacher-Masoch wrote a novel in 1870 about sexual submission. From him, we get the word *masochism.* Leave it to Sigmund Freud to pull it all together, in 1905, and create the word *sadomasochism.*[29] At the time, Freud, thought engaging in such behavior was neurotic, but times sure have changed. Engaging in BDSM can be as simple as spanking, being tied up, or wearing a blindfold or handcuffs and can go all the way up to sex swings and sex dungeons. There can also be role-playing and acting out BDSM fantasies.

Before you go *Grey*, it is important to have a conversation with your partner about what's going to happen and set clear boundaries on the things that you are okay with and those that you are not. As much as *50 Shades* gets wrong about the real world of BDSM—from the types of ropes you and your partner should use to the manipulative, abusive tactics the characters employ—one thing that it gets right is that a lot of trust and open communication is required to engage in any acts of kink or BDSM. In many cases, one partner dominates the other, who is the submissive. Often the submissive will be immobilized or blindfolded while the partner touches, strokes, bites, pulls hair, or spanks. The submissive is totally giving up control and can't initiate any contact, but can only respond to what the partner is doing. Use your imagination as well as ice cubes, feathers, or a vibrator on your partner. There aren't hard-and-fast rules about what you can or can't do except for those that you mutually agree on before you begin. One thing you should make clear is a word or phrase that lets your partner know to stop what they are doing.

If you and your partner discover that BDSM could be more than just a blindfold and some light spanks on the behind for the two of you, there are plenty of kinky individuals who would likely welcome you into their community. There are Web sites and clubs that connect like-minded responsible adults that you can find online if you only start to look.

TOYS AND OTHER JOYS OF SEX

Sex toys can add another level to your pleasure, either when you are getting off by yourself or if you are with a partner. You can buy products online, at the drugstore, at your local retailer, or at a sex shop. You may feel inclined to shop in solitude—no need to be embarrassed!—but going shopping with your partner either online or IRL can add some anticipation to your play as you browse through toys, explore, and discuss which ones may be fun for you two to share. There are toys that vibrate, toys that simulate penises, toys for clitoral stimulation, toys that will stimulate you both at the same time, toys with remote controls, toys you can sync with your cell phone, toys for anal play, and everything from nipple clamps to furry handcuffs. No judgment—whatever works for you for solo play or for you and your partner together, as long as you both agree on when and how the toys will be used, is great. A few popular items include:

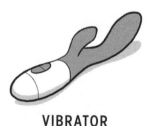

VIBRATOR

The trusty vibrator—you may have one resting in the top drawer of your beside table right now. What's great about vibrators is that there is one for everyone. They come in every color of the rainbow, all shapes and sizes, all levels of intensity, and at all price points so that you can choose the one that suits your needs and your body. The song says diamonds are a girl's best friend, but many women are not so sure about that.

The Rabbit

These dual-action vibrators are shaped like a penis with an extension shaped like rabbit ears, which are perfectly placed for clitoral stimulation so you can get your vibe on internally and externally at the same time. Some rabbit vibrators have a rotating feature in the shaft for extra stimulation.

Vibrating Bullets or Eggs

These little powerhouses can up your pleasure. Small and discrete, they come in a wide range of shapes and sizes that you can use with or without a partner. Some have remote controls that can be used from a distance to get you tingly while your partner quite literally pushes your buttons. There are also vibrators that the two of you can use simultaneously.

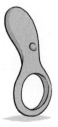

COCK RING

This little toy is a flexible ring that goes over his penis and sits toward the base. It serves to restrict bloodflow to keep him harder longer and delay orgasm. Some rings come with a vibrator for extra stimulation.

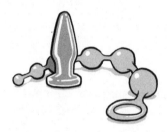

ANAL PLUGS AND BEADS

These toys will enhance your anal play. Use them alone or use them when you are having sex to stimulate an even bigger O—for either him or you. It's best to start small with these and work your way up to larger toys. And don't forget to lube, lube, lube!

On the less sexy side, when shopping for sex toys it's important to think of them as an investment in your pleasure and to comparison shop and read reviews before you buy. Medical-grade silicone is the best material for toys, because while it can be a bit more expensive, it is much easier to clean and really cuts down on any risk for bacterial growth. Other materials are hard plastic, jelly rubber, cyberskin, glass, and stainless steel. With all toys, it is best to use water-based lube so it's easier to clean up; use condoms; and don't put anything in your anus and then in your vagina without cleaning or covering the toy with a fresh condom.[30]

Be sure to clean your toys on the regular and follow the manufacturer's instructions. Obviously, if they have a motor and batteries, unless they are waterproof, you don't want to be submerging them in the sink or loading them in the dishwasher, although some toys are top rack safe! A washcloth with soap and water is usually the best way to clean them—and they should be cleaned after every use. You may even consider giving a clean to your toys *before* you use them to be sure they are free of any germs or bacteria they may have picked up from the drawer in your bedside table. Speaking of storage, keeping your toys in a clean cloth bag is usually the best way to prevent them from being damaged as well as keeping them clean. If your toys are made of porous material (hard plastic, elastomer, thermoplastic elastomer or TPR, or jelly rubber), they can still have bacteria on them after a wash, so use a condom if you are sharing.

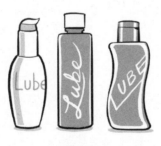

LUBE

Everybody can use lube, and there is a lube for everybody: water-based lubes, silicone lubes, organic lubes, and lubes scented or flavored. There are kosher lubes and vegan lubes. There are lubes that are appropriate for any lifestyle and activity. That's a lot of lube choices.

Make your va-jay-jay happy with lube! Because the skin and tissue of the vagina can be sensitive, it really is best to go hypoallergenic and avoid scents and flavors. Save scents for massage oil that will only be used externally, and maybe try out a flavored lube for when you go down on your dude.

Check your labels. You want to avoid glycerin, propylene glycol, polyethylene glycol, petroleum, parabens, benzyl alcohol, and citric acid. These additives can lead to irritation of the vaginal area and can also foster yeast infections or UTIs. Watch out for benzocaine, which is a numbing agent that is added to some lubes to counteract pain and often used for anal sex. Hey, if it hurts (and not so good), you should probably not be doing it, as you are numbing the nerves that would let you know that you are tearing the sensitive tissues in your body.

These are the three main types of lubes:

WATER-BASED

While they don't last long, can be sticky, and can't be used in the shower, water-based lubes are really the best for vaginal sex. They are fine for use with sex toys, no matter what material they are made of, and they will not cause any damage to condoms. They are easy to wash off and won't stain sheets. You might just have to keep the container handy beside the bed and add more when you need it!

NOT FOR LUBE

There are a few things that may seem as if they would be a good substitute for lube if you run out, but they are a no-go for when you are having sex, some because they can degrade condoms and others because they just don't work or are simply not a good idea.

Coconut oil. Can make the latex in condoms deteriorate, rendering them useless for preventing pregnancy or sexually transmitted diseases.

Crisco. We're sure you have some around the house, but it shouldn't be used around your vagina. It could cause irritation, and it also will be bad for latex condoms.

Spit. Usually not slippery enough and could lead to spreading an STD/STI.

Vaseline. Not a good candidate for lube: Not only can it mess up latex condoms, it can also potentially cause an infection.

Baby oil. It is oil, so it's the enemy of latex condoms, but it can also upset the useful bacterial in your vagina and leave you with a yeast infection.

Lotion. The risk with lotion is that it may have additives and perfumes that would be lovely on your skin but might cause irritation in your lady parts.

In general, it's best to stick with commercially prepared products to smooth the way toward satisfying sex.[31]

SILICON-BASED

Great for vaginal sex, as well as anal sex, silicon-based lubes are superslippery, last a long time, and can be used for sex play in the shower or bath. You should know that they can damage silicone toys. They can also stain, so be forewarned!

OIL-BASED

Oil-based lubes are best for masturbation, as they have a thick consistency and are often less irritating to sensitive skin. They can damage latex condoms and cause them to break down or tear, making them useless for pregnancy protection and for preventing STDs or STIs. Be careful with oil-based lubes, as they are more difficult to wash off than other types of lube. And if they get inside your vagina, they can stick around (literally) and become a magnet for bacteria, which can lead to an infection, so they are best not used for penetrative sex.

Sex is not just one thing or one behavior. Lucky for you, no matter how you express yourself sexually, your vagina is equipped to receive all types of pleasure from self-stimulation to toys to penetrative sex. That's because your V is uniquely designed so it can get itself ready for action by becoming wet with its own form of lube to accommodate everything from a finger to a penis to a dildo. Pretty impressive.

5

STAYING HEALTHY 101: KEEPING YOUR VAGINA HEALTHY AND HAPPY

A HEALTHY VAGINA IS a happy vagina. Having a healthy, happy vagina means a healthier, happier you and, here's the big plus, super sex! This chapter will clue you in on all aspects of the care and feeding of your vagina from health foods for your vagina—yes, what you eat can influence the health of your vagina—to what to expect from your gynecologist visits. It's important to know what's normal or average and what might be a problem when it comes to what can happen in your vaginal vicinity, so we'll walk you through some of the more common health-related issues that arise, how to recognize them, and what to do about them as well.

GOING TO THE GYNO

First things first: A gynecologist is a medical doctor who specializes in the care of women, particularly of their reproductive organs, and an obstetrician is someone who cares for women during pregnancy, childbirth, and postpartum. Many doctors have training in both specialties, and that's where we get ob-gyns. There are a number of ways to find a doctor. You can search on your health insurance Web site for doctors in your area who take your plan, you can ask friends if they have recommendations, you can check out doctor-rating Web sites, or you can ask your primary care doctor for a referral (you have one of those, right? You should.). You can also go to your local Planned Parenthood or health clinic. Your doc should be board certified, and it's a good idea to know what hospital she is affiliated with for future reference in case you need a hospital for a health issue or for giving birth. Find out if you will always see the same doctor—whether she's there part- or full-time—or if you will see other doctors in the practice. Find out when the office is open (hours and days of the week) and if it offers late-night or early-morning appointments that might work best for your schedule.

GROOMING FOR YOUR GYNO

Your gyno doesn't care if you shave your legs, groom your pubic hair, or even if you have your period, but she does care that you are honest about your sexual activity and any troubling symptoms you may be having.

PLANNED PARENTHOOD

Planned Parenthood is a nonprofit that, through its clinics, provides inexpensive reproductive health care services to women in the United States through funding from the federal government, private insurance co-pays, and donations to the organization.

How Planned Parenthood is funded has been a contentious issue in the United States for quite some time. The services that Planned Parenthood provides to women (and men) are largely preventive and diagnostic. They conduct STI/STD screenings, provide contraceptive advice as well as contraceptives, give pregnancy tests, give Pap tests (for cervical cancer screening), and provide abortions. The fact that Planned Parenthood provides abortions is the bone of contention over funding, particularly from the federal government. However, abortions make up a small percentage of the services they provide, and abortions cannot be paid for from the funding the organization receives from the federal government.[1]

Despite the controversy, these clinics continue to provide care to women across the United States.

If you are seeking the care of a private doctor covered by your insurance, most doctors will be willing to set up an appointment so you can meet them and decide if you want to be their patient. When you go to the office for the meeting, you are not just evaluating the doctor, you are really trying to get a feel for the whole practice. Is the waiting room nice? Is the receptionist friendly and informative? Did they call you back right away? When you speak to the doctor, you want to assess how easy she is to talk to and how she responds to any of your questions. Is she thorough? Dismissive? Did she answer the question you asked? Is she judgmental? Remember, if you decide to get your care from her, the next conversation the two of you have will be with you naked, apart from a paper gown, your feet in stirrups, and she will be looking at your personal parts. This is someone you want to feel comfortable talking with about your body and sexual behavior.

Once you have decided on a doctor, you should see her annually. If you have insurance coverage, most plans cover annual "Well Women" visits, which is a euphemistic name for gynecologist visits.

WHAT HAPPENS AT AN APPOINTMENT?

In the exam room, you will remove all your clothes and put on a paper or cloth medical gown, open to the front. You might want to leave on socks because you will be putting your feet up in stirrups, and they can be cold!

If it's your first time with the doctor, she will probably run through a medical history with you, which will include your personal medical history as well as that of your family—primarily your parents. She'll be looking for any history of cancer, including breast or uterine, and history of heart and cardiovascular disease. To get a sense of your overall medical background and health issues, she'll probably ask about major illnesses, hospitalizations, and any vaccinations that you have received. She will cover questions about allergies and childhood illnesses. She will ask about tobacco, alcohol, and drug use—past and present. She will want to know if you are taking any medications and if you are under the care of another doctor, including a primary care physician or other medical professional like a therapist or psychiatrist. She will also want to know if you are taking any supplements, as those can interact with birth control or other medications. Essentially, she is trying to get a sense of your overall health and any risk factors you may have. She will ask you about your period. She'll want to know when your LMP (aka last menstrual period) was, how regular you are, and if you have any problems when you menstruate, including severe pain or excessive bleeding.

She will ask about sex. It seems obvious, but it's important to tell her your sexual history with as much information as you can provide. She is totally not there to judge, she is there to get to know you and the behaviors that can have an impact on your overall as well as reproductive health. It is important to be honest with her about when and what type of sexual activity you have engaged in, especially if you have had unprotected sex, meaning sex without a condom. She'll want to know how many partners you have had as a way to gain understanding and perspective on your sexual behavior and health—again, no judgments.

In an appointment, some basic health assessments will be taken, including height, weight, blood pressure, and temperature (these may be taken by a nurse or tech). Your doctor will likely conduct a breast exam and will want to know if you do self-exams or need information on how to conduct a self-exam.

Depending on your age and medical history, she may refer you for a mammogram to screen for breast cancer.

Next, she will want to check the health of your vulva and vagina. You will be lying on an examination table with your feet in stirrups—a footpad or extension from the exam table that allows your legs to be up in the air so your doctor can have a clear view of your vulva and vagina. She will examine the vulva to look for signs of infection or irritation. She will then use a speculum, a metal or plastic device that your doctor inserts into your vagina to hold it open while she conducts her examination of your vagina and cervix. If you are getting a Pap test—used to check for cervical cancer—she will use a long-handled brush to collect cells from your cervix that she will send out for testing. She will insert her gloved fingers into your vagina and push on your abdomen to feel your cervix, ovaries, and uterus. This can be a little uncomfortable, but it doesn't take long. If you are being tested for sexually transmitted diseases (STDs), she may do the blood draw in the office (usually done by a nurse or a tech person), or you may need to go to a lab to have the blood taken and tested and your doctor will give you a prescription to do so. You may be asked to use the restroom to pee in a cup, because urine color and odor can be indicators of gynecological health. Your pee may be tested in the lab for blood cells, protein, sugars, and other measures that can indicate an imbalance or disorder. Your doctor will talk to you about birth control so you can determine if you want or need birth control as well as what form would be best for you, your lifestyle, and your health.

An important part of the appointment is when she asks if you have any questions. This is when your mind will likely go blank. It can be helpful, if you do have any concerns, to write them down on a card or put them in your smartphone prior to your appointment so you don't walk out of the office and say, "Oh, I forgot to ask…"

Issues that women commonly bring up in an exam are:

- Period irregularity
- Pain during periods
- Pain during sex
- Lack of interest in sex
- Bleeding after sex
- Unusual odor or discharge from the vagina
- Potential side effects of birth control that is being prescribed
- Desire for a new type of birth control

It bears repeating here: Your doctor has seen a multitude of vulvas, vaginas, and cervixes; has heard a huge range of sexual experiences of many women; and has seen and treated myriad vaginal issues. Keep in mind, she is a professional and is there to help you and keep you healthy, so being fully open and honest is the best way to go. She is also someone to speak with if you have been sexually abused or assaulted, because not only can she assess any health repercussions, she can point you in the right direction for other resources or treatment. If she is operating as your primary care physician, then she can give you a referral to other doctors.

In the normal course of events, you will see your gyno once a year for a checkup and diagnostic tests (as needed).

GYNO, PRIMARY CARE PHYSICIAN, OR BOTH?

Do you need to have two doctors—one for gynecological issues and one for everything else? The answer is: It depends. Many primary care physicians (PCPs) can conduct pelvic exams, breast exams, and do Pap tests and other gynecological tests. Many gynecologists also measure your blood pressure, listen to your lungs, and ask about general health issues. A lot depends on you and your doctor. If you have a primary doc who does Pap tests, you may be set up for one-stop shopping. If you go to a gyno who asks about your overall health and well-being, you may also be set. It can be helpful for your doctor to know if she is the only doctor you are seeing for all of your health monitoring and treatment. If your PCP feels you need to see a gynecologist, or if you get pregnant and need to see an OB, then your PCP can refer you. Likewise, if your gyno sees that you have a funky mole, she may refer you to a dermatologist. The thing is that your vagina doesn't exist separate from your body, and the health of the vagina is influenced by your overall health, so you do want to work with someone who is looking at the big picture of your health as well as focusing on your vaginal and reproductive health. Whatever way you can get the best care possible for you—with one doc or two—is the way to go.

Cancer Screening

Cancer of the cervix can be detected by assessing cells of the cervix. The test used is a Pap test, aka Pap smear. You should have your first Pap by age 21 and then receive one every 3 years. Once you reach age 30, you can be tested every 5 years for HPV and Pap together. Other cancers your doctor will be concerned about are breast cancer and ovarian cancer. (Your doctor will do a manual breast exam and may refer you for a mammogram. There is no definitive test for ovarian cancer, but if you have symptoms like bloating or pelvic pain, speak with your doctor.)

STDs/STIs

Even if you are in a long-term, monogamous relationship, your gynecologist will speak with you about STDs and infections because it is possible for STDs to linger in your system and be dormant for many years. Get tested so you can be sure that you (or your partner) haven't picked up something along the way. Don't let what happened on your junior year abroad or at that crazy concert come back and haunt you. STDs/STIs can be tested via blood or urine sample. Whether or not your doctor orders testing depends on risk you are exposed to and any symptoms you may have. See pages 204–211 for more information on STDs/STIs.

KEEPING YOUR VAGINA CLEAN AND HEALTHY

An annual visit to the gyno is a good practice for keeping tabs on your health. However, there is much you can do the other 364 days of the year for the care and upkeep of your V. You don't have to go to heroic measures because the vagina itself is pretty amazing in the cleaning department: It is an essentially self-cleaning organ. Sorry to put an image of your vagina as a self-cleaning oven in your head, but it really is pretty self-sufficient. Left to its own devices, your vagina doesn't need much help staying clean, and the labia and vulva only need a daily cleanse with some plain, gentle, unscented soap and water to get rid of sweat, skin cells, menstrual blood, or any urine that you may not have removed with toilet paper.

CLEANSE CAREFULLY

Soaps with scents and excessive chemicals can irritate your skin, cause rashes, and leave you super uncomfortable with itching or irritation. Liquid body washes and soaps can have ingredients like alcohol and sulfates that your skin may find irritating and should be avoided for use in the genital area. You really want to keep it simple with a mild bar soap and use a washcloth or your hands when you clean yourself off in the shower. Skip the mesh shower puff or loofah, as they can scratch

BUBBLE, BUBBLE, CAUSING TROUBLE?

Rumor has it that taking bubble baths can cause yeast infections. We say this rumor is not *exactly* true, but taking a super soak in the tub with your favorite scented bath bomb can get rid of the infection-fighting bacteria in your vagina—the good kind of bacteria that you want to keep around. So should you only take showers? Nah, go ahead and have a bubbly bath, but be sure to not linger too long, and completely rinse off all the soap when you are done and then towel-dry.

the delicate tissue and leave you open to irritation or infection.

After having sex, you may feel like you need a super cleanup what with all that lube and whatnot in your nether parts, but your usual routine will be just fine to clean up your labia and pubic hair. Again, your vagina is self-sufficient in the cleaning department, and no extraordinary measures are needed. (See also "To Douche Or Not To Douche?" on page 191.) If you have anal sex, be sure your partner washes up and/or changes the condom before having vaginal sex, as the bacteria in the anus can lead to an infection in the vagina.

FLOURISHING FLORA

The vagina itself has healthy bacteria—called lactobacillus— that can be disrupted by too harsh a cleaning regime, allowing bad bacteria to flourish. Bad bacteria leads to itch and infections. Additionally, the vagina has an acidic pH that may prevent overgrowth of those other bacteria that can lead to even more infection. You don't want to do anything to upset that delicate, and protective, balance. Unless you have some sort of infection, you don't need to help the vagina to keep its pH in balance by using any wipes or creams, no matter what the advertisements tell you or how happy the lady looks on the box. Really, your vag is a-okay on its own. Be aware that taking antibiotics can upset the balance of the vaginal flora in your vagina, so be sure to eat extra yogurt that includes *Lacobacillus acidophilus* and limit sugar intake when on these medications.

Another strategy for keeping that vaginal flora healthy is to use condoms, which also seem to help keep the pH balance in the vagina where it needs to be.

SO FRESH AND SO CLEAN

If you are prone to UTIs, you might want to look into getting a bidet, as it can help wash away bacteria both before and after having sex. If a bidet isn't accessible or possible, a handheld showerhead can do the job. T.P. is still the best for post pee or poo, though!

FERMENTED FOODS

As we have mentioned previously, your vagina doesn't operate all on its own: Its health is connected to your overall health. Because the positive bacteria in your vagina is influenced by what you eat, it is important to eat things like cultured yogurts to maintain the proper balance. Lacto-fermented vegetables also can promote healthy bacteria in the intestines and throughout your system. Sources of these health-promoting probiotics include yogurt, kombucha, kefir, sauerkraut, and kimchi. Or you can check with your doctor about probiotic supplements.

Other foods that can be great for vaginal health include:

- Green tea: Can help fight UTIs.
- Omega-3 fatty acids found in fish like tuna or salmon: Have anti-inflammatory properties that may help with period cramps.

- Soy products (edamame, tofu, tempeh): Have a compound in them that mimics estrogen and can combat vaginal dryness.

One note here: Do not put food in your vagina. Despite what some old wives' tales say, putting something like yogurt, a clove of garlic, or tea tree oil in your vagina to deal with a yeast infection is only going to be messy, potentially cause additional irritation, and could promote an infection rather than cure it. Also, we don't care how phallic that cucumber, carrot, or banana looks, or how "sexy" putting whipped cream or chocolate on your labia may seem to be, do not put any food products in or near your vag. You could be introducing bacteria or damage your delicate skin. Any of these foods could lead to upsetting the natural pH balance of your vagina. All of which could trigger a nasty yeast or bacterial infection or, at the least, uncomfortable irritation. Not a good idea. Leave the fruits and vegetables on your plate and keep them away from your passion pit.

BREATHABLE BRIEFS

No matter what type of undies you wear, from granny panties to thongs, if you can go with cotton, that is best for your vagina and surrounding area. Cotton allows your lady parts to get some air and can also absorb moisture. Tight workout clothes or nonbreathable undies can lead to vaginal discomfort, so try to find underwear and workout clothing that absorbs or wicks away moisture. You want to avoid dampness between your legs, because excess sweat can inspire yeast and bacteria to grow. Yeast loves warm, damp places. If you really want to air things out, go commando—but maybe not when you are wearing those brand-new stiff jeans, as your crotch area can get irritated and scratched. If going commando during the day isn't your thing, then go commando at night in a nightgown or loose-fitting pajamas so you can air out your vulva.

WICKING WORKOUT WEAR

Keep your vaginal area covered at the gym for workouts. Even if you are wearing leggings or shorts, don't go commando there, as you could pick up bacteria from benches or exercise equipment. Additionally, underwear can help wick the sweat away from your vulva and labia, keeping them from getting too damp. A caveat: As much as no one wants a visible panty line, a thong is not the best choice for workouts. It can move back and forth as you exercise, whether you are doing yoga sun salutations or sprinting on the track, and can transfer bacteria from your butt to your vulva. Not a pleasant thought or a pleasant feeling later.

When you hit the locker room, put a towel down on the bench when you get out of the shower or keep your towel wrapped around you to avoid contact with a seat that may have bacteria on it. Also, if you are not showering immedi-

YONI MASSAGE

Now you can get a personal massage for your vagina. Known as a yoni massage, its purpose is not to achieve orgasm—it's not really like those massage happy endings you've heard about—but to find and release sources of tension in your vulva and vagina, depending on your level of comfort, with the goal of improving your ability to orgasm. If you go for a yoni massage, be sure your masseuse uses gloves and clean hands and speaks to you about what is happening so you can consent before she touches. Also, some yoni massages come along with steam cleaning and herbs—you may want to skip the steam, as you could get burned, and the herbs may be irritating, so your yoni may end up saying "yee-ouch."[2]

ately, try to change out of your sweaty workout clothes as soon as you can. Sitting around in damp clothes if you run off to meet friends after exercise class can cause irritation of your vulva and labia. This advice also applies to wet bathing suits. Sitting around in them can promote a yeast infection. We are not kidding when we say that yeast really likes those warm, damp places, so change or dry yourself off thoroughly or you run the risk of getting itchy and infected.

If cycling is your workout of choice, either outside or at your gym's or cycling studio's spin class, be sure to wear padded bike shorts to keep the pressure off and protect your genital area. If you are wearing padded bike shorts, then you can skip underwear, because the pad is created to protect your genitals as well as wick away moisture. We know it sounds a little strange and it may feel weird at first, but it is the best way to get the most out of the padded shorts and protect yourself from injury. If you feel pain or numbness in your crotch from bike riding, try tilting the nose of the seat up slightly, which will shift your weight off your genitals and onto your sitz bones. Or you can try using a wider seat. Be sure the bike is set up properly for your size. For an outdoor bike, have a bike shop help you adjust the fit so the seat height and handlebar placement are correct for you. At your cycling class, ask the instructor if he or she has recommendations on setting up the bike to avoid any issues. If any numbness in your crotch lasts for more than a week, time to spin on over to your doctor to get things checked out.

SIMPLE SANITATION

Cleaning up after you pee is pretty straightforward. Toilet paper will do the trick, but be sure to wipe front to back so you don't introduce any fecal bacteria into your vaginal area. And your back door is wiped front to back as well, keeping any poo away from your urethra so you won't develop a UTI or worse. Toilet paper should be unscented to avoid irritation. Some women love to use bidets for a fresh, clean rinse, but toilet paper is truly a better choice (unless you are prone to UTIs— see pages 222–224). You may wonder about using feminine

---

TO DOUCHE OR NOT TO DOUCHE?

Let us put it this way: No. Douching will wipe out the all the bacteria in your vagina (good and bad) and completely upset the bacterial and pH balance, putting you at risk for infection or disease. If you are worried about odor and want to douche to get "clean smelling," you need to speak with your gyno about what may be causing the odor. It is normal to have a slightly musky vaginal scent, but if you notice a change in your odor and it becomes foul or fishy, check in with your doc. A douche can mask any odor that may be there, but it will also mask the ability to find the underlying cause of the odor. Besides, whoever said your genitals should smell like tropical flowers? Plus, there is potentially an increased risk of ovarian cancer from douching, and you don't want to mess with that.[3]

---

wipes. They are likely fine, but be sure that you choose alcohol-free, glycerin-free, and fragrance-free to avoid potential irritation or reaction.

FORGO FADS

There is a current trend happening of "steam cleaning" the vagina. It is definitely not something you should do. There is no evidence it does any good, and there is a big risk for burning your lady bits. Ouch! Stick to steam cleaning your face, not your fanny. And here's another fad: How about a wasps' nest in your vag? Sold as "oak galls" with the promise of tightening up, cleaning your vagina, and reducing discharge, the ground-up wasps' nests are inserted into the vagina to do their magic. Um, no. Just no. We advise examining trends like these with a skeptical eye and reading up on science-backed benefits of products and therapies before taking any risks that you could end up regretting.

Any itching, burning, or discomfort you experience in your vulva, labia, or in your vagina should be discussed with your doctor. It may be that you need to switch soaps or change up your cleaning routine, or you may need treatment for an infection.

THE HAIR DOWN THERE

We are mammals and we have hair. In fact, one of the first signs of sexual maturation is hair growth in the armpits and pubic area. Ironically though, after all that fuss we kick up about wanting to be grown-up, one of the first things we all try to do is make the hair go away. Hair is completely natural, but cultural aesthetics influence how much we tolerate hair, particularly in the pubic and bikini line area. Everyone has their own level of comfort with how much or how little hair they can deal with, and that can change over time. Some women leave the hair natural and don't cut or trim at all—rocking the "bush." Some take off enough hair so it will not show when wearing a bathing suit or bikini, usually around the tops of the thighs, aka "the bikini line." Some remove all but a little patch of hair—the "landing strip" look—while other prefer to take it all off and leave only smooth skin behind, otherwise known as a "Brazilian."

How you want to deal with your grooming is all up to you. Before you start razoring or tweezing, lasering or waxing, remember that the skin in that area is very delicate, and hair can serve as a form of protection for your tender skin. If you decide to reduce or remove the hair near your vagina, you need to be gentle to your skin and be aware that hair removal can sometimes lead to irritation or ingrown hairs or other issues. There are a variety of hair-removal methods, so you should be able to find the best way that works for you.

Hair removal can be DIY or done at a spa or dermatologist's office. No matter how you remove the hair, you want to be kind to your skin to prevent further irritation or bacteria growth afterward. Post–hair removal, you should wear loose-fitting clothes for the rest of the day, have no sun exposure for 24 hours, and avoid sex or vigorous physical activity for 12 to 24 hours, again to avoid irritation.

There are enough methods for removing hair that you can find one that is right for whatever body part you'd like to address. You can take the hair off your legs, arms, eyebrows, and face, too, all with their own risks and ideal methods, but we'll be focusing on the vaginal area here. Some hair-removal methods and products can be irritating to skin, so check labels if you are allergic to any cosmetic ingredients or products.

With creams, lotions, and waxes, it would be a good idea to test a small area before you get the product near your lady bits to assess your skin's response. You don't want to eliminate the hair and gain a nasty allergic reaction in its place. Read all instructions carefully.

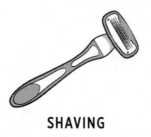

SHAVING

Although quick and relatively cheap, the downside to shaving is that you run the risk for nicks and cuts as well as ingrown hairs. Don't shave dry! You can use water, soap and water, or shaving creams or gels to allow your razor to move smoothly over your skin. Many razors also have lubricating strips to help with potential irritation. Taking it slowly can help you avoid nicks and cuts—beware the knees, shins, and ankles! You can discourage ingrown hairs by *gently* rubbing the shaved area with a washcloth after defuzzing or, if you have the time, exfoliate before shaving. Applying lotion to your skin following your close shave can also help to soothe and moisturize. Don't use a disposable razor for more than a week—they are disposable for a reason, so toss and always work with the sharpest blade possible.

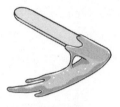

WAXING

Removing hair with hot wax can be done at home or at a salon. In the salon, the hot wax is applied to the hair, then a strip of cloth is pressed onto the wax and is pulled off, removing the hair and its root. FYI, and full disclosure, it hurts! Like, hurts! But some women feel the temporary pain is worth it to get a hair-free area. Book the appointment during the 2 weeks following your period, because the week before you get it you will more sensitive to pain. When you are at the salon, make sure they are using new wax for your treatment and that there is no "double-dipping" going on—a fresh applicator stick should be used each time wax is applied. This will help avoid introducing bacteria into the area. There is a risk for burns if the wax is too hot, and the process can irritate skin.

You can get waxing kits at your local beauty supply, drugstore, or pharmacy. The at-home kits have wax that you warm up in the microwave, then apply to the skin and pull off or remove with fabric strips. There are also preloaded strips that you warm between your hands, place on the skin and hair, and pull off.

Your skin can be irritated after any method of waxing, so following the hair removal you can apply some soothing lotion or oil—home kits typically come with an aftercare lotion—and wear loose clothing. Waxing can last for 4 to 6 weeks. It is best not to wax if you are taking tretinoin (Retin-A) or isotretinoin (Accutane), as you can be prone to skin irritation while on these medications.

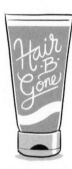

DEPILATORIES

These hair-removal creams, lotions, or foams can be found in your local drugstore or pharmacy. You apply the product to the area where you want to go bare, it dissolves the hair shaft, and you wipe or wash away the remaining product, taking the hair with it. Some products come with a plastic blade for smooth removal of hair. Read labels carefully, as you don't want to use a product intended for your bikini line on your face, and vice versa. Hair removal can last for 3 to 5 days, then you'll need to repeat. It might be a good idea to spot test the option you intend to use before you apply it all over, just to be sure you don't have any sensitivities or adverse reactions to the chemicals in the depilatory.

ELECTROLYSIS

Typically performed by a professional, this process involves a tiny needle directing an electric charge into the hair follicle to destroy it. Depending on where you live, practitioners offering electrolysis have varying requirements for licensure or certification, so you should check credentials before you make an appointment. At the very least, they should have some accreditation and work in a clean space, use gloves, and answer all of your questions about cost, the number of treatments you will need, and how long each session will last. Electrolysis will give you permanent hair removal.

There are devices that you can purchase at stores and on the Web that will allow you to do electrolysis at home or that use a heated wire to get rid of hair. DIY with electricity near your girl parts just doesn't sound like a great idea to us, but you can try it. Just know that some of these devices can lead to injury or damaged skin, so if it's your first venture with electrolysis, perhaps it's best to go with a trained professional.

LASER

A medical procedure that is done in the dermatologist's office to disrupt hair growth, lasering basically kills the root of the hair so it won't grow back. If it does, it comes back lighter and finer than before. Lasering treats a larger area than electrolysis can. There is a risk for burning or skin damage, so be sure to go to someone who is licensed for doing the procedure. It takes several treatments to get full hair removal, and each treatment can be expensive. Once you have had the full set of treatments, the removal can last for years, but you may need annual touch-ups for the best results.

Now that you have the lowdown on how to get rid of the hair down low, the question becomes how much should go? The answer is totally up to you. Culturally, there seems to be a negative bias toward pubic hair, assuming that it is somehow dirty or unattractive. So, many women opt to go hairless. Reasons for doing so range from feeling like it makes sex more sensual or that their partner is more likely to perform oral sex. Porn is definitely an influence, as most women in porn go bare. Bottom line on the bush is to trim, shave, or remove as much or as little as you'd like, but when you do so, be gentle to your skin and see a dermatologist if you develop a rash or irritation that doesn't go away.

TATOO TABOO

If you want to get tattoos, stick to other parts of your anatomy, as the skin near your vagina is supersensitive and could become inflamed or irritated by the tattoo process or have an angry reaction to the dye in the tattoo.

WHAT YOUR VAGINA IS TELLING YOU

If only your vagina could talk. Or maybe not, depending on what you've been up to. But if you are going to take the best care of your vagina, you will need to pay attention to any signs your vagina may be sending you about its health.

With the sheer amount of product devoted to masking or eliminating smells coming from your nether regions, you would think that the vagina would be surrounded with a constant cloud of stank unless you take aggressive action. Truth is, the vagina smells like a vagina, and everyone has her own particular scent. If you notice a strong or unusual odor that you have not had before (especially if it comes along with an itch or if you feel burning when you pee), you should talk to your doctor about it. Trying to cover it up by using scented wipes or lotions or sprays could potentially make things worse by causing further irritation or delaying effective treatment. Some say that eating to maintain a healthy gut microbiome can help with your scent. The idea is to avoid sugar, dairy, and coffee; to load up on green leafy veggies; and to eat yogurt and fermented foods so that your overall microbiome and in turn, the microbiome in your vagina, will be healthy and in balance.

DISCHARGE

We've said that the vagina is set up for self-cleaning, and part of that cleaning process is discharge. The discharge comes from glands in the vagina, and the purpose of discharge is essentially to carry away bacteria and dead skin cells and to keep the vagina clean and moistened. Usually discharge is white or clear and can have a watery or sticky consistency depending on the time of the month and your cycle. Around midcycle, it can be slippery and stretchy, and this consistency of discharge usually happens when you are ovulating. Isn't it nice that your vagina can tell you when it's "go time" for baby making? It's the vagina's way of preparing an easy-access path for sperm to make its journey to an egg for potential fertilization.

Although most women assume any itch in their panties is due to a yeast infection, before you self-diagnose and run off to the drugstore to treat it with an over-the-counter remedy, it's really best to see your doctor. Using the wrong OTC medication can prolong your agony as well as allow whatever is going on to get worse. Your doctor can ID the offender and give you a prescription or guidance on the proper course of action to resolve the itch.

Other types of discharge that you should be aware of and that most likely require a doctor's exam and evaluation are listed beginning below.[4] Remember, if you notice something going on with your discharge, turning to Dr. Internet for a diagnosis isn't the best health choice. See a real doctor so she can examine you, ask questions, and possibly take a sample of the discharge for testing to determine what's going on and how best to treat it.[5]

White, Lumpy, and Comes with an Itch

The most likely scenario here is that you have a dreaded yeast infection caused by a fungi known as candida, which can be brought on by antibiotic use that disturbs the normal flora of your vagina or by sitting around in sweaty workout clothes—that'll teach you to go straight to brunch after yoga without switching out of that damp underwear and those tight leggings. Same for wet bathing suits. Pregnancy, diabetes, and birth control can be triggers for a yeast infection. It is not caused by having sex. While there are some effective over-the-counter treatments for yeast infections, you should see your doctor first

---

YEAST INFECTIONS GONE ROGUE

Yeast infection is typically due to a fungus called candida, but it is also helped along if the balance of your good bacteria to bad bacteria is out of whack. So yeast infections can show up on places other than your va-jay-jay. The good news is the treatment that works for vanquishing yeast in your vag (like an oral med or antifungal cream) will work in other places as well. If you scratch that itch even though you know you shouldn't, you run the risk of spreading the infection to your butt!

Unrelated to your vaginal yeast infection, you can also get a yeast infection on your feet, commonly known as athlete's foot. If you have diabetes or are immunosuppressed, you can get it on your skin. Dudes can get itchy from yeast on their penises, and an antifungal cream will clear it up. Note that he won't "catch" a yeast infection from you if you have one. He would likely get it from the same perfect storm of sweat and warm, damp clothes that triggers most overgrowth of candida/yeast, just like you did.

to be sure that it truly is a yeast infection you are dealing with. Your doctor can prescribe an antifungal that should clear things up, or she can recommend an over-the-counter treatment, as that can also be effective in vanquishing a yeast infection. On the whole, yeast infections are relatively easy to cure.

Thin, Watery, Grayish, White, and with a Fishy Odor and Possibly Itchy

Bacterial vaginosis (BV) is a common cause of vaginal discharge and is usually accompanied by intense itching. It is triggered by the pH balance in your vagina being thrown off by anything from diet to tight clothes to not adequately cleaning your genital area. When the pH of your vagina gets out of balance, that allows for the overgrowth of a normally occurring bacteria, gardnerella, which will overwhelm the good bacteria. Douching, IUDs, and multiple sex partners can also contribute to your getting BV, and BV can lead to other health problems like pelvic inflammatory disease (PID) (see page 221) as well as make it more likely to get infected with HIV (if exposed; see pages 208–209). Your doc can prescribe an antibiotic to treat the infection.

Yellowish Green Cloudy Discharge

This can be due to the STDs/STIs chlamydia or gonorrhea (see pages 204–205). Chlamydia is spread through oral, anal, or vaginal sex and is caused by bacteria. If you are sexually active with more than one partner, you should be tested for chlamydia regularly. Another fun fact about chlamydia is that it can be symptom-free, so if you are sexually active, you should get tested even if you feel okay. Gonorrhea is caused by bacteria and is spread through all forms of sexual contact. Both of these STDs/STIs can be treated with antibiotics. Your partner should be tested and treated as well. To be sure not to spread these STDs/STIs, you need to use a condom during sexual activity.

Frothy, a Little Smelly, Grayish/Greenish

This could be trichomoniasis, a common STD/STI that you don't actually have to have sex to get. All the pain without all the fun. It's caused by a little organism that can lurk in vibrators, towels, and other objects. So be sure to clean and disinfect sex toys, and don't use other people's towels (after they have used them). Because it can be transmitted by sexual contact, be sure to use condoms when you have sex. Trich can be treated with antibiotics.

Blood

If there is blood in your discharge, sometimes right after your period is finished or right before it starts, it could be that the blood was slow to clear out of your vagina from previously menstruating and it's not something to worry about. If, on the

---

THE CLAP

The sexually transmitted disease, gonorrhea, is also known as "the clap," and it is unclear why. A likely explanation is that an old French word for brothel, *clappier*, is the source.

other hand, you see blood in your panties and you are sure it's not your time of the month, then you should speak with your doctor. Some women can "spot" because of birth control, vigorous sex, being pregnant, due to an IUD, medication, or illnesses like thyroid disease or PCOS. In any case, crimson in your underwear when it is not your time of the month is a situation that you should have a professional check.

WHAT YOU SHOULD KNOW ABOUT STDS/STIS

STDs/STIs are more common than you might think. And you don't have to do the walk of shame every day of the week to get one. Someone you know has probably dealt with one of these infections at one time or another. Maybe you have. Unfortunately, there is a lot of guilt and finger wagging that gets piled onto having an STI, but many are simply infections that can be vanquished with antibiotics, so where is the shame in that? Is it

---

STD OR STI?

Is it a sexually transmitted disease (STD) or a sexually transmitted infection (STI)? The two terms essentially mean the same thing, but *infection* has less of a stigma than *disease*, and many health-care professionals are using the term *STI* because it feels less judgey and is a more accurate description of conditions like chlamydia or herpes.

really any different from any other antibiotic-treatable infection?

At the risk of repeating ourselves, the best action to take regarding preventing sexually transmitted infections is to practice safe and mutually consensual sex. Also, if you have engaged in unprotected sex, get tested by your doctor to be sure you are in the clear. Be sure your partner has been tested, too!

We mentioned chlamydia and gonorrhea on page 202, which are both sexually transmitted diseases that will often, but not always, signal they are active by changes to your vaginal discharge (potentially along with itch or burning when you pee). A number of other sexually transmitted diseases pose varying degrees of health risk that can linger in your system or recur. The best prevention (have we mentioned this?) is to have protected sex with a condom of your choice every time you have sex.

Although we are primarily focusing on the vagina, don't forget that STDs can be passed through oral sex as well. Bacteria and viruses can move between your vaginal and anal areas to your mouth via sexual contact as well as through semen and blood. You can prevent herpes, HPV—which causes oral cancer—gonorrhea, and chlamydia from infecting your mouth by using male condoms, female condoms, and dental dams during oral sex.

Along with a Pap test, get tested annually for STDs/STIs as well as for HIV if you are sexually active. Also, if you've already had an STD/STI, don't think you are off the hook for future infection or testing. Unfortunately, you can contract a different STD/STI or have a recurrence of an old STD/STI. Safer sex and getting tested on the regular are the way to go to keep from getting an infection or having one come back with a vengeance.

GENITAL WARTS

Caused by a virus, these warts can appear soon after contact with an infected partner, or they can take some time to show up—2 to 3 months after infection. They vary in appearance, so if you see any growths on your genitals that look like a fleshy colored bump or look a bit like cauliflower, have your doctor check it out. You can't get rid of the virus once it's in your system, but the warts can be removed by freezing them or using a prescription cream. Sometimes they even clear up on their own. And remember what we said about condoms being great for preventing STDs? Well, they are generally, but in the case of warts, condoms are not foolproof. The virus can lurk beyond the area that a condom covers, so any skin-to-skin contact can pass it on. The HPV vaccine (for women up to age 26) can protect you from the viruses that lead to genital warts.[6, 7]

HEPATITIS B

This viral infection that can affect the liver is spread by contact with infected blood or body fluids via sexual activity, needles, or blood transfusion. There are two other hepatitis viruses—hep A and hep C. Hepatitis A is most often spread through food that has been contaminated with feces either in water or by being handled by someone who did not wash their hands properly after going to the toilet. It's one of the reasons why every bathroom in every restaurant you have ever been in has a sign that says, "Employees must wash hands." Hepatitis

C is mostly spread through blood. There are vaccines for A and B, but no vaccine for C.

HERPES

There are two types of herpes and, to be completely honest, a huge chunk of the world population is infected. According to World Health Organization researchers, an estimated 3.7 billion people under age 50 are infected with HSV-1, the cause of cold sores, and for HSV-2—the STD—another 417 million people worldwide ages 15 to 49 have it. But interestingly, 140 million adults have genital infections caused by HSV-1, meaning half a billion people could sexually transmit either virus. Spread through skin-to-skin contact during vaginal, anal, and oral sex, the sores that characterize herpes can start as a reddish bump that is superpainful, then they can ooze and crust over. You can have outbreaks on any part of you from either strain.

A doctor can diagnose you through a physical exam, a culture, or a blood test—but it's worth noting that the Centers for Disease Control and Prevention (CDC) does not recommend testing asymptomatic patients for the disease, as nothing can be done when you are not showing symptoms. Although there is no cure, and the virus stays in your system forever, antiviral medication can reduce breakouts, help manage any pain, and lower the potential spread of the infection. Keep in mind, just because the sores are not "active," it doesn't mean that you can't spread infection. Have your partner wrap it up for sexual activity to prevent spreading the virus. Many women get herpes breakouts when they have their periods. Note that there is current research into a herpes vaccine that would reduce outbreaks.[8]

While there is a lot of stigma surrounding herpes, it is worth recalling those staggering statistics about the number of people who are infected and remember you are not alone.

Also remember that this disease doesn't destroy your sex life unless you let it. Communication, medication, and condoms can help.

HUMAN IMMUNODEFICIENCY VIRUS (HIV)/ACQUIRED IMMUNODEFICIENCY SYNDROME (AIDS)

First off, HIV and AIDS are not the same thing but are often discussed together, so we'll clarify the differences here. Human immunodeficiency virus (HIV) essentially attacks the white blood cells in your blood so they can't defend your body from bacteria, viruses, and other infections. In other words, HIV knocks out your immune system and opens you up to potentially contracting a host of infections that can attack you body's systems. When HIV has destroyed enough of the lymphocytes, or "T cells," and they reach a low level in your bloodstream, then you will have acquired immunodeficiency syndrome (AIDS).

Infection occurs through exchange of blood, semen, and vaginal fluids. This can happen through sex, sharing contaminated needles, or being stuck by a contaminated needle by accident, as could happen to a doctor, nurse, or other health-care worker. Because the disease was initially diagnosed in gay men, it was assumed that they were the only population who could contract the disease and it was considered to be terminal. We now know neither is the case. There are men and women around the world who have HIV or AIDS, and there have been great strides made in treating and managing these two diseases. Although there is still no cure, and in some countries the drugs are difficult to obtain, each is now considered to be a chronic disease that can be treated with medications.

The best prevention against contracting HIV/AIDS is safer sex by using a condom. That, and not sharing needles with anyone if you are taking intravenous drugs. If you are a health-care worker, be sure to follow all protocols for safely handling bodily fluids as well as needle management and disposal.

Testing for HIV is done through a blood test. It's a good idea to be tested if you are not sure if you have had contact with someone with HIV, if you have had multiple sexual partners, or if you are planning to become pregnant, as HIV can be passed to a baby during pregnancy, childbirth, or breastfeeding. If you are going to have sex with a new partner, ask about the person's health history and use a condom until you can be sure you are both free of STDs/STIs.[9]

HUMAN PAPILLOMA VIRUS (HPV)

Human papilloma virus is, sadly, incredibly common. Seventy-nine million Americans currently have it, with 14 million new cases expected each year. It can lead to developing warts or genital warts (see page 206), and some forms of HPV can lead to cervical cancer. HPV is spread by skin-to-skin contact. While it is always a good idea to wear a condom to prevent the spread of infectious disease, a condom doesn't guarantee you won't get HPV. However, if you are age 26 or under, you can get the HPV vaccine, which is delivered in a series of three shots spaced over the course of several months. Although many have questioned the effectiveness of this vaccine, the CDC recently conducted a study that showed HPV rates for teen girls and women in their early twenties have dropped dramatically since the vaccine became popular in 2009. Speak with your doctor about being vaccinated if you haven't already been.[10, 11]

PUBIC LICE OR CRABS

These little critters, also known as crabs for their crablike appearance, attach themselves to pubic hair and potentially other hair on the body, where they lay their eggs. They feed on your blood, and their bites can become very itchy. An infestation of pubic lice can be extremely irritating and possibly lead to a skin infection. Because the lice are usually transmitted through sexual contact, it is possible to have STDs/STIs at the same time as when you have crabs. Treatment can include applying a cream with 1 percent permethrin to the pubic hair and then combing out the nits (eggs) with a fine-tooth comb. Bedding and recently worn clothing should be washed in hot water, and any recent sexual partners should be notified so they can seek treatment. Once treated, you should be in the clear, as the lice will be eliminated.

SYPHILIS

This STD is caused by the bacteria *Treponema pallidum*. If you contract syphilis, you will develop a painless ulcer about 3 weeks after you have been exposed that will then ooze and release bacteria that can be spread by sexual contact via vaginal, anal, or oral sex. The sore can heal, but you remain infected, because without treatment syphilis is a lifelong disease. The earlier it is treated the better, because syphilis is a progressive disease. The first stage is when you get a genital sore, which can resolve on its own after a few weeks. In the second stage, which can last about a year, you can develop a rash, fevers, or fatigue. The next stage has no symptoms, but you are still infected. The final stage, about 10 years after first exposure, can lead to damage to your brain, organs, and spinal cord—and ultimately, death. You doctor can diagnose syphilis with a culture of fluid from an active sore and/or blood tests. Having syphilis can predispose you to being susceptible to HIV, so if you test positive for syphilis you should also get tested for HIV. Treatment with antibiotics (typically for you and your partner) at the early stage can cure syphilis. At later stages, antibiotics can halt the progress of the disease but not repair any damage that may have already occurred. If you have syphilis, at any stage, you should wear condoms when you have sex.

WHEN YOU KNOW, HOW DO YOU TELL?

We're going to be honest here: Sharing the news about having an STD/STI is not going to be easy, but it is oh so very important to do it. Opening up about such personal information will need to be done in your own way, and in your own time, but don't wait for the stars to align before you let a partner or potential partner know about your condition. You may want to practice what you will say with a friend so you can get used to hearing yourself talk about your STD/STI. For a past or present partner, you need to tell them soon so that they can be tested before they put anyone else at risk. When you are ready to tell a potential partner, although it may seem easier to do so over text, it may be better to have an in-person conversation. Also, timing is everything; don't wait until you are about to get up close and personal to say, "Before we go any further, you should know…" Depending on your partner, they may need some time to digest your big reveal, and it will likely require further conversation about what it means for your relationship. The key thing is to be open and honest, and to practice safer sex.

You may find yourself in a situation where you have been diagnosed with an STD/STI but do not know who gave you the disease. Once you have been diagnosed, it is important to let any previous sexual partners know about your diagnosis, because sometimes an STD/STI can have no symptoms or can take some time to reveal itself. Your previous partner or partners who may have been exposed should seek out a doctor so they can get an exam and get tested. They need to know not only so they can seek treatment but also so they alert their present and current sexual partners about getting tested and treated and know to practice safer sex to avoid passing on the STD/STI. It might be an awkward conversation. You might find yourself face-to-face with a few angry exes that you never wanted to see again, even under happy circumstances. But their health is on the line, and you do the right thing by informing them.

WHEN SOMETHING IS OFF . . . WOE DOWN BELOW

As noted on the previous pages, you don't have to have an STD or STI to experience pain or unusual discharge or develop growths or irritation on the skin of your genital area. In fact, there are a number of fairly common conditions that you don't need to freak out about but that should probably spur you to check in with your doctor so you can get the right treatment.

WHY DOES IT BURN WHEN I PEE?

And when we say "burn," we mean feeling like you are peeing tiny little razors or broken glass—maybe both at the same time. Although a burning sensation when you pee can be an indicator for an STD, it is quite possible that it is a urinary tract infection (UTI; see pages 222–224), or that you simply have irritation from having sex. The skin around your vaginal opening can get tiny tears or abrasions from sexual activity, so when you pee it can feel the same as when you get lemon juice on a paper cut. Ouch!

ACNE

Yep, those pimples don't only pop up on your face and back—they can show up down south, too. Having vaginal acne is annoying but not a problem. Don't pick or pop (same goes for anywhere a pimple shows up), keep the area clean, and possibly try products with tea tree oil or natural antibacterials to help clear up the skin. Bacterial buildup can lead to acne developing and can be due to prolonged time in sweaty workout clothes or not washing up properly. Shaving can also bring on infected hair follicles, so if you are having recurring acne, give the complete deforestation of your bush a rest and see if things improve. If you are applying a product to deal with the acne, after you check with your dermatologist or doc on what is best, use it only on the exterior of your vulva and not on the more delicate skin of your inner labia.[12]

BARTHOLIN'S CYST

On either side of the vaginal opening are glands that are responsible for lubricating the vagina called Bartholin's glands. If one of these glands becomes blocked, then fluid can accumulate in the gland and cause swelling, which will feel like a little lump on one side of the opening to the vagina. It's not particularly painful and can usually be relieved by soaking in warm water or using warm compresses. If it gets super-painful, releases pus, or you don't feel well—as in you have a fever or chills—go see your doctor. The gland may have become infected or need to be drained, and you may need a round of antibiotics to clear it up.[13]

BLEEDING

Of course you are going to bleed when you get your period, but bleeding at other times can happen as well. It's common to "spot" or bleed between periods when you are on birth control. You can spot sometimes when you are pregnant. You can also see some blood after sex. Post-sex bleeding can be due to damaged delicate tissues of your vag or it could be the sign of an STD/STI or—in severe cases—it can be a sign of cervical cancer. If you bleed or spot once in a while, no worries. If it happens frequently, then have a word with your gyno to be sure all is good.[14]

BOILS/ABSCESSES

It sounds like some ancient biblical curse, but you can develop boils in your vaginal area. Usually they are due to whatever you have been using to remove the hair down there. Boils can build from razor bumps, ingrown hairs, or infected hair follicles that fill with pus. Change your razor blades often to prevent introducing bacteria to your skin when you shave. Don't pick or poke the boils, as you could spread an infection. A warm compress can provide relief, as can wearing loose underwear and clothes to keep pressure off the blisters. They should clear up on their own, but if you get a fever and they don't go away, see your doc.[15]

CONTACT DERMATITIS

When is irritation, burning, and itching not an infection? When it is contact dermatitis. This irritation of the skin can be caused by anything from laundry detergent to shower gel to feminine hygiene products like tampons with deodorizers. If you have recently changed the soap you use in your shower, switched your laundry detergent, or started using new condoms or a new type of lube, one of those might be what is causing the itch. Stop using the suspected product and see your doctor so she can rule out or confirm that it is a skin irritation and not some form of infection. Contact dermatitis can even be triggered by shaving with a dull razor or friction from sweaty workout clothes. In addition to using a fresh razor and changing out of your workout garb once you are done, the best approach is to use hypoallergenic soaps, lotions, and cleansers. If you have a latex allergy, it could be triggered by condoms, so be sure to use condoms that are latex-free. Contact dermatitis can be cleared up with a topical cream prescribed by your doctor and with home care like soaking in a lukewarm bath. To keep it from recurring, use perfume-free, additive-free mild soap on your body as well as in the laundry.[16]

CYSTITIS

Cystitis is an infection of the bladder that can cause inflammation and irritation. Indications of cystitis include pain when peeing, abdominal pain, and feeling as if you have to pee more often than usual but not peeing much when you do go, as well as smelly, cloudy urine. Cystitis happens when bacteria gets into your urethra, which goes up to the bladder. Bacteria can be pushed toward the bladder by sexual intercourse. Frequent sexual intercourse can sometimes lead to bladder infections, which is why cystitis is sometimes called "honeymoon cystitis." You will be diagnosed with a urine sample and then put on antibiotics. The same preventative measures for UTIs (see pages 222–224) apply here, such as wiping front to back, peeing after sex, and drinking cranberry juice.[17]

DRYNESS

If your lady parts are dry as a bone and making you itchy, know that this situation can be common in perimenopause or menopause but can also be triggered by medications like antihistamines. Your dry itch can kick in right before your period when your estrogen levels go down, causing your skin to become irritated and parched. Additionally, low-dose estrogen birth control pills can make your vagina less lubricated. All of this dryness not only can make you itchy and but can make sex uncomfortable and make you more likely to suffer tears in your delicate areas. The best approach is to use an over-the-counter vaginal moisturizer that is free of additives, perfumes, and so on, but if the problem persists, then it's time to get it checked out by your doctor. She may change your birth control or prescribe an estrogen cream to get some moisture back in your vag.[18]

ECZEMA OR PSORIASIS

These two disorders cause rash and itching of the skin, and your skin down below is not exempt. Psoriasis is an autoimmune condition, and eczema is usually caused by the skin overreacting to an irritant. So if you know you have either of these issues and you end up being itchy in your panties, eczema or psoriasis is the likely culprit. A mild steroid cream can help alleviate the itch, but check with your doctor for the best approach. Carefully evaluate any over-the-counter medications before applying them to be sure they will be suitable for use on your vulva or labia.[19]

ENDOMETRIOSIS

You can experience pain, particularly during intercourse, if you have endometriosis, a disorder that causes the tissue that is normally inside your uterus to grow outside of your uterus (see pages 149–150). It can feel like the pain is in your vagina, but the true source is usually found during an exam by your doctor to be pain in your abdomen. Painkillers and hormone therapy can help.

FIBROIDS

Fibroids, which can run in families, usually develop when a woman is in her thirties or later. These common, noncancerous growths occur in the uterus or outside the uterine wall and can make PMS cramps seem like a walk in the park. We're talking serious pain here. You could also experience heavy periods, back pain, and the need to pee often as a result of fibroids. Your doc can diagnose them with an ultrasound or an MRI and, depending on their size and where they are located, she will remove them surgically. There are some hormonal medications that can shrink the fibroids, but these tend to have symptoms similar to menopause and are tough to tolerate.

ITCH

As discussed, there are many sources of itch on your vulva and vagina ranging from yeast infections (see pages 200–202) to STDs/STIs. If your skin is just a little dry (as can happen in winter) or if it is irritated from shaving or wearing tight clothes, you can do a little DIY de-itch with a mild product like petroleum jelly or coconut oil—as long as you are only using it on exterior skin, not putting it inside your vagina or around the vaginal opening. If the dry skin doesn't clear up, see your doctor to be sure it is not an infection requiring treatment.[20]

INJURY

A bump, a bruise, a burn, a scratch can happen anywhere on your body, so it should come as no surprise that you can injure your hoo-ha in these same ways. Bruises are uncommon but can happen from slammin' sex (literally) or if you slip on your bike and hit that crossbar (major ouch!). Most bruises will clear up over time. You can get burned from wax that is too hot, so be careful when you wax away hair on your own, and ask to test the temperature at the salon as well. You can tear your labia if you are too dry when you have intercourse or use a sex toy or if sex is a bit rough. You'll know, because you may have pain, blood, or it will hurt when you pee. Using lube can help avoid tears, but if you get one, it will usually heal on its own.[21]

INGROWN HAIR

That waxing, shaving, and plucking can have more consequences than simply baring your skin. Curly pubic hair can curl back into the skin and form a bump that can become pus filled and tender to the touch. An ingrown hair is not a big deal, but it can be painful, and because the skin of the vaginal area is so delicate, it must be treated gently. Usually ingrown hairs resolve on their own, but an ounce of prevention can keep those ingrown hairs away. Keep the area clean before you defuzz, and use a washcloth gently after hair removal to exfoliate and liberate any stray hairs that may take a turn for the worse. Don't pick at the ingrown hair. Try products with glycolic and salicylic acids that will disinfect and help unclog the hair.[22]

LICHEN SCLEROSUS

If you get white spots on your vulva that itch like crazy, it could be that you have lichen sclerosus, also called "eczema of the vagina." A buildup of white plaques that thin the skin caused by hormonal imbalances or autoimmune issues, lichen sclerosus should send you running—or carefully walking—to your gyno for a diagnosis, where you can get prescription medication to find relief, usually steroids or topical estrogen.[23]

ODOR

As previously discussed, unusual odor coming from your vaginal area could be the result of an infection (see pages 202–203) that should be evaluated by your doctor. Other sources of odor coming from your vagina could be a forgotten tampon or even a condom that slipped off your significant other and stayed stuck behind. Be sure to remove tampons or other products when your period is done.[24, 25]

PELVIC INFLAMMATORY DISEASE (PID)

With this infection of the uterus, ovaries, and/or fallopian tubes, you may feel some low-level pain or discomfort, but it is something that should be treated, because scarring due to PID can impact your fertility. Sometimes an untreated STD/STI can lead to the infection, so if you have any questionable pain or discomfort, speak with your doctor so she can evaluate you and get you started on antibiotics to clear up the infection. PID can act up when you get your period; if you spike a fever when Aunt Flo is visiting, see your doctor.

SYRINGOMA

These little pimplelike flesh-colored bumps are caused by the sweat ducts near your vagina clogging up. Syringomas can also erupt on the face and around the eyes. They are harmless and usually resolve on their own. Some people are more prone to developing syringomas than others. As with anything that shows up on the skin of your vulva or labia, it is best to get it checked by your doctor to determine the cause as well as the best course of treatment.[26]

URINARY TRACT INFECTION (UTI)

This all-too-common unwelcome visitor drops by when bacteria—typically E. coli—gets into your urethra—aka the opening you pee from—and makes its way to your bladder. The bacteria can get there through improper wiping or sex, so keep yourself clean by wiping front to back and making sure your partner doesn't touch or put anything in your anus and then your vagina. Make sure your sex toys are clean, too, and remember you can always use a condom on them and change the condom if you are inserting into a different body part to keep things clean. When you get this infection, your urinary tract swells up, making you need to pee more and making it painful to pee, and causing pain in your pelvic area. If you think you have a UTI, don't hesitate to go to the doctor. If left untreated, you can develop a kidney infection, so it's best to get on antibiotics as soon as possible. Antibiotics are the only way to banish the bacteria that is making you miserable. Ironically, antibiotics can also be the cause of UTIs. As you know, antibiotics are used to get rid of infection-causing bacteria, but they are so good at the job that they take out good bacteria, too, leaving you with an imbalance in the health of your flora in your intestines as well as your vagina. Any time you are on antibiotics, give your flora a boost with probiotics or eat more yogurt with live cultures.

Also, when you get to the doctor quickly, she can determine if your symptoms truly are the result of a UTI or caused by another issue like an STD/STI. Good practices you can follow to minimize UTIs and avoid reinfection are:

- Do take all of your meds, even if you are feeling better.
- Don't have sex while the infection is active to allow the infection and inflammation to get better.
- Don't use sex toys while you have a UTI, and if you are prone to UTIs, consider not using toys in your vagina at all. The irritation may be provoking infection.
- Drink lots of water (we know, peeing may not feel pleasant, but you want to keep hydrated and flush out your system).
- Don't hold it in, either, as that may exacerbate the problem by keeping the bacteria in your bladder. You need to pee.
- Eat and drink foods with vitamin C (or take vitamin C supplements).

Some natural supports for when you have a UTI are oregano essential oil capsules and D-mannose supplements. (Always talk to your doctor if you are taking a prescription medication and also want to take an herbal or other supplements to be sure there are no potential problems or interactions.[27])

A few things can lead to further irritation of your bladder. If you can cut back or avoid alcohol, artificial sweeteners, coffee, and spicy or acidic foods or drinks while you have the

UTI, it may help you feel better. We're sure you have heard that old wives' tale about cranberry juice helping relieve UTIs. Well, surprise! It turns out it's true! As long as it is 100 percent natural cranberry juice, drinking it may help ease your symptoms.[28, 29, 30]

Now you have the recipe for a healthy V: good hygiene, safer sex, wiping correctly, keeping sex toys clean, avoiding lots of perfume or deodorizers, not using harsh chemicals or soaps, getting some air down there, wearing cotton panties more often than not, and checking with your doctor if something doesn't smell right, look right, or feel right. Better to check it out than let an infection or other issue go untreated, because you can become more seriously ill or, in the case of infectious diseases, spread the disease to others. Nobody wants that.

6

SAFETY 101: HARASSMENT TO RAPE—WHAT YOU NEED TO KNOW

JUST BECAUSE YOU HAVE a vagina, it doesn't mean that you are a delicate flower that needs to be protected—quite the opposite, actually. Women are perfectly capable of taking care of themselves, *thank you very much*, but to do so you need to know potential safety pitfalls, your rights, and what to watch for so that you can speak up for yourself as well as advocate for others. We're all in this together, and sisterhood—humanhood—can keep us interacting with one another in a respectful way that promotes safety at home, in the workplace, and beyond.

If you feel like all of this talk about responsibility sounds like we are letting guys off the hook and that the burden for making change falls on women's shoulders, don't misunderstand. Men need to check their behaviors, take responsibility for their actions, and speak up for the women and girls in their lives if something is going on that shouldn't be. We won't lie: Nothing is more attractive than a guy who says he is a feminist and instead of mansplaining to us about women's rights, he listens to what we need and want and acts as a true ally. But since this book is primarily for women, we'll be looking at these issues through that female lens, addressing what women can do to tackle these issues in their lives.

The sad reality is that sexual harassment and sexual assault are issues faced by women on a daily basis. Although they are never the victim's fault, it is worth learning how you can keep yourself safe, respond appropriately, and educate those around you.

SEXUAL HARASSMENT

Sexual harassment can happen to anyone, and it can happen pretty much anywhere and anytime. It can happen in the workplace, at school, or out on the street. It can happen in the gym, in the grocery store, or at a bar or restaurant. You get the idea—there are really no safe zones.

STREET HARASSMENT

Sadly, most women have experienced "catcalling"—random strangers on the street making comments that more often than

---

"SMILE, SWEETHEART!"

Smiles are often viewed as a requirement for women. No matter whether she hasn't had her morning coffee yet or it's late after a long day, a woman who isn't smiling will find herself constantly reminded that she is failing to meet societal standards. To add insult to injury, she is reminded to smile by some total stranger on the street. When a man tells a woman to smile, what he is essentially saying is that she needs to change her appearance to please him, regardless of her emotional state. And we are just not having that. While we are at it, can we move that the whole concept of "resting bitch face" be retired? Sure, scientists have proved it's a real thing,[1] but guys have it, too, so the whole name is just sexist. Why must women be labeled bitches if they aren't smiling? Let's not grin and bear this one any longer.

---

not are sexual. In fact, a recent study that surveyed 16,000 women in 20 countries—the largest study of its kind to date—has shown that a shocking 84 percent of women have been harassed on the street before they even turn 17.[2] That girls are experiencing such an invasion so young is heartbreaking. This "attention" can be anything from whistling to graphic comments about a woman's body or what the commentator would like to do to her. Many a woman has experienced the feeling that simply walking outside invites the comments of every Tom, Dick, or Harry, of being treated like public property when she is simply on her way to work, running errands, meeting friends, or going home. It doesn't seem to matter the time of day or the attire a woman is wearing. Although, of course, what she is wearing is often given as an excuse or the subject of the comments. Simply being on the street often makes a woman fair game to some men. A lot of guys—and some women—will say that this attention is positive and it's a compliment to be noticed. They will insist: "Why would you be upset when someone thinks you are hot? It's a compliment." But for the majority of women, it feels like a violation and makes them uncomfortable, objectified, and angry. It can also be embarrassing and intimidating.

Being catcalled can get especially uncomfortable when a woman doesn't react the way the harasser wanted, which is to respond with "Thank you" or to treat the verbal assault as a compliment. Then the guy might start calling her out for being a bitch or being stuck up, or he straight up changes his mind and now yells at her that she is ugly. It can be scary. As annoying as this situation can be, because it usually happens in public and

---

CARDS AGAINST HARASSMENT

If you have ever wanted to make a clever comeback to someone who is harassing you on the street with catcalls, but you've come up empty, these cards are here to come to the rescue. Created by a young woman, the cards explain that a woman being outside walking around shouldn't be subjected to comments from random strangers. They essentially tell the guy to STFU, but in a creative and intelligent way. Check them out here at www.cardsagainstharassment.com/cards.html.

on the street, you can simply keep walking and ignore the dude who thinks he is doing you a favor by telling you have a nice ass. Besides, you will probably never see him again. If a guy starts following you and continuing to go off, it's time to enlist help by either entering a store and asking for help or getting the attention of those around you, then calling the cops.

The situation gets trickier when a woman knows the person making inappropriate comments and/or has to interact with him on a daily basis.

HARASSMENT IN THE WORKPLACE

It seems like every time we turn on the television or read the news, there is yet another story about a celebrity or bigwig CEO, board member, or boss who has been sexually harassing women in the workplace. Awareness is out there—many employers require training and have strict policies in place to protect against sexual and nonsexual harassment as well, covering race, religion, or comments that are demeaning or discriminatory— but it doesn't mean the situation has been resolved and that someday you won't find yourself on the receiving end of unwelcome comments from a boss or coworker.

Your workplace may well hold a comprehensive seminar or training program on what sexual harassment is, lay out the company policy concerning sexual harassment, and provide information on the avenues to report a problem, but unfortunately, many women don't report an issue for a range of reasons.

Sometimes they don't want to cause a problem or be seen as a troublemaker—after all, they would be reporting their boss, and that would put them in an uncomfortable position, and they worry they won't be believed or that they will lose their job. People can sometimes start to second-guess themselves and, as time goes on, may begin to believe that they did something to attract the attention. We've all heard of so many "he said/she said" situations where what she says is not believed, or she is told she is exaggerating or that she "can't take a joke," that it's easy to understand why someone may hesitate before escalating the issue.

The odd comment from a boss or coworker probably won't fall under harassment, as the harassment needs to be extensive or severe to be actionable. Sadly, that one comment probably won't be the last, and the unwelcome remarks or behavior will likely get worse over time. If a male colleague notices or says something about your new haircut or clothing, telling you how nice you look, it is most probably sincere and meant as a compliment. If he wonders aloud what your hair looks like after a night of sex, he's crossed the line. Especially if he does it consistently. It's the persistence of his perverse comments that should send you to human resources (HR). That and if he gets physical and grabs or pats your butt or other body parts. Also, if he is your boss or in a position of authority and straight up says, or hints, that you will be rewarded on the job, in terms of a raise, promotion, more interesting work, or a better assignment, if you have sex with him or engage in sexual behavior, that should send you to HR.

Note that although most sexual harassment is older male to younger female, it can also be same sex, and the ages and genders can be reversed. If someone is talking dirty to you, making sexist comments about you, putting their hands on you in a way that is uninvited, making inappropriate comments, or sending inappropriate images or e-mails to you and any or all of this behavior makes you uncomfortable, you need to speak up.

Sometimes the lines are not completely clear. What if someone makes an off-color joke? What if you don't agree about what is, or is not, offensive? In the case of behavior or comments being up to interpretation, your company policy should lay out what is acceptable and what is not acceptable in the office or workplace. You can go to your boss with concerns or questions. You can let the person know that you don't like that type of joke or that you find what was said offensive. They may not tell that type of joke or make those comments in your presence again, which is great, but if they continue because they know it bothers you, then there is a real problem.

We all know someone who has had an office romance, so what happens when coworkers flirt with one another? Does this mean that there is no room in this world for dating someone from the job? Not at all, although you may want to check your company's policy regarding dating in the workplace before getting involved with a coworker. The flirting that happens in a relationship that starts on the job is usually mutual and doesn't cause either party discomfort or make them feel unsafe at work. Although we will caution that if things don't work out, you will need to see and work with this person after the breakup, which could be awkward—something to take into consideration before things go too far.

So what do you do if a boss, coworker, or client is harassing you? The best approach is to be calm and firm and tell them,

"Please don't talk to me like that. I find it offensive." Or "Please don't touch me like that." It's important that you make it clear that their language and behavior is unwelcome. Laughing it off or saying nothing can be interpreted as going along with the interaction. Then go back to your desk and document the who, what, when, and where of what has just occurred. Use as much detail as possible regarding the language the harasser used. If the behavior continues, add the subsequent incidents to your document; then you will have something specific to take to human resources. You want to be able to demonstrate that the way this person is treating you is a pattern that has continued over time and has made your work environment uncomfortable, if not hostile. While *hostile* may sound like a strong term, you don't want to spend your days at work wondering if he is going to make some lewd comment or cause you to feel discomfort or embarrassment. It's difficult to do your job well when you are stressed about something like this.

It's important to make a complaint to HR with your documentation. It is their responsibility to put a stop to the behavior and protect you from the unwanted attention. And if the situation requires that you go beyond the workplace for it to be resolved—in other words: lawsuit—you will have documented the things he has said and done to you if you choose to speak to a lawyer.[3] (See Resources for links to further information.)

Workplace Bullying

Being hassled at work isn't always sexual harassment—you may simply be bullied. Unfortunately, many women find themselves in this situation on the job, and the sad news is that they are often the victim of another woman. So much for solidarity in the workplace! The boss who steals your ideas, belittles you in front of colleagues, yells, insults you, and does so on a regular basis is a bully. Being bullied is a terrible situation to be in because—on top of feeling completely beaten down and insulted—it can seem as if there is nothing you can do, particularly if it is someone who is a direct boss or your superior.

Although it can be difficult to keep your cool in the middle of a barrage of bullying, you can try to defuse situations by weathering the storm and focusing on discernable, actionable work-related issues that are being thrown at you amid the abuse and let the boss know how you will solve those problems. Try to keep coming back to these issues during your interactions. If you are being sniped at by a boss or colleague—as in she ignores you, belittles you, humiliates you in front of others, cuts you out of meetings, or engages in the type of behavior that gives you flashbacks to the mean girls of middle school—you can calmly speak to her and ask her to stop what she is doing. Calling her out on her behavior may be enough to get her to lay off. If, in either case, nothing changes, then you can go to HR—with the same sort of documentation of what's been going on that you would bring in a sexual harassment situation—and sit down to try to talk through the issue and find a solution. Bullying is not illegal, but HR may be able to step in and clear the air between you and a coworker, and they should be able to intervene if a boss is mistreating you. If the situation is so bad you need to change teams or positions, you will need HR's help.

HASSLED WHILE WORKING OUT

If you run or walk for exercise, you have probably experienced the same sort of catcalls that many women receive for simply being out in public. It's unpleasant at any time, but you may feel more vulnerable when you are wearing workout clothes and someone catcalls or makes comments about your appearance. The best approach is probably to ignore the person and continue on your run or walk. Keep an eye out for your surroundings and note where you can change your path to disconnect if someone continues to hassle you or make comments. There are those who tell women never to run alone, but following that advice can set up a roadblock to your ability to exercise if you can't find someone to go with you. Besides, you may enjoy running or walking solo. You need to decide for yourself what is safe. Yes, you should be able to exercise outside without fear of being bothered, but there are creeps out there, so keep an eye out and remember your safety is more important than getting in that last mile of your run. Keep your phone with you so if you need to call for help or just to let a friend or partner know where you are, you can.

In the gym, you may receive unwelcome comments. Some people will say that you are trying to get in shape, so what's the big deal if someone makes a comment about the body you are obviously working so hard to get to look good? Well, much depends on how that comment makes you feel, how often it happens, and if the attention is unwelcome. Because the commenter may be someone who you see on the regular because your gym schedules are the same, it's worth responding with a "Please don't say that. It makes me uncomfortable." The person may go on the defensive and claim the comment was only meant as a compliment. But if you are polite and hold your ground, you should be okay. If the person persists, then you can speak to the gym management about it. This approach of deflecting and then reporting also goes for an instructor who is inappropriate with language or touch. Certainly, personal trainers or instructors likely need to touch you to adjust your alignment or form while you are working out or to make comments on your body or fitness, but there is a difference between positive reinforcement for the work you have done and a comment that has a sexual connotation. You will also know if they are making physical contact to correct positioning or of they are lingering in that contact unnecessarily. If you don't say something, it is likely to continue. If, when you do say something, the person continues to be inappropriate, then you need to speak to their manager. Silence can invite continued behavior. It does seem unfair that the burden to address the situation falls on your shoulders— why doesn't anyone tell these people what is and isn't appropriate behavior?—but if you don't speak up, it won't stop.

HARASSMENT ONLINE

If your workplace and gym are chill and everyone respects one another, then you are in a very good place. But let's say that after dodging dudes on the street asking you to smile, you reach the sanctuary of your home and find that your phone is blowing up because your ex posted those tasteful nudes you took for him on Reddit when he was out of town. The breakup wasn't super bad, but he clearly is still pissed and is trying to hurt you online. Welcome to the world of "revenge porn." Know that if he posts naked images of you without your permission, that is called nonconsensual porn. Yes, porn. Sadly, there are sites that post revenge porn, and your photos and information may appear on these public sites without your permission. Explicit photos and images can be offered for sale on marketplaces on the Dark Web. Even worse, some sites will ask for a fee to take down photos posted without your permission—which is illegal, not to mention repulsive. Unfortunately, if the information or images go viral, the damage has probably already been done, as the naked or explicit pictures of you may have already been seen by multiple people—including employers, friends, colleagues, and family members.

If you are the victim of invasion of privacy, revenge porn, or online harassment, you should consult with a lawyer to see what steps you can take—laws vary state by state regarding these issues. In the meantime, it is best to document what has been put out there with the URL of the site, the date, and as much information as you can put together, including screen shots or printouts of the material. Your instinct will be to try to delete it, ignore it, and hope it will all go away, but it won't. Having backup and all the information documented will help if you pursue legal action, and it will also be valuable when you take action to get the information taken down from any relevant Web site. Web sites have varying policies on content that they will not allow or that they will take down, so you'll likely need to reach out to each site's administrator individually.

While it can be easy to walk on by if someone on the street catcalls you, it is much harder to walk away if the harassment is online. A troll who makes a nasty comment on a public forum is easy to ignore. But someone who is targeting you can reach you

ONLINE BULLYING—WHAT TO DO TO MAKE IT STOP

If someone is heaping sexist, racist, threatening abuse on you on Twitter, Facebook, or Instagram, here are some steps to take.

- Take screenshots of their statements so even if they take down their posts, you have proof.
- Unfollow them or block them.
- Report the abuse to the host site.
- If there are threats of violence, contact your local police.

Another approach for documenting online abuse is to go to HeartMob, a site where you can report abuse and ask for assistance and advice (https://iheartmob.org).

Sometimes it is hard to determine who is doing the bullying online, as comments and posts can be anonymous or are put out under a pseudonym. Often, disengaging with that particular poster can stop the problem: They, like most bullies, want to get a reaction, and if their actions don't achieve the desired effect, they move on. But it is always best to report the bullying so that the offenders can't just target their next victim. If you speak up, you may save someone else from the type of bullying you experienced.

via e-mail, Facebook, Twitter: anywhere and everywhere you use social media. Because being connected is usually an essential part of your work and your social life—you can't completely disconnect from the Internet to get away from someone who is harassing you—you have to take swift action. If you are the victim of stalking, sexual harassment, or threats via e-mail on social media, you should document the material and report it to the company where the material appears (like Facebook, Twitter, etc.) as well as speak with your local law enforcement. Local laws vary, but it's worth reaching out to the police so that you have documentation of the threats and the issue. Should you need to seek out a restraining order, you will have materials to back up your request.[4] (See Resources for sources of information on the practical and legal issues for dealing with abuse online.)

ABUSIVE RELATIONSHIPS

Time to get super obvious, but it bears saying: No one should ever hit you, punch you, push you, grab you, or physically abuse you. No one should ever scream at you, constantly criticize you, demean you, or verbally abuse you. A healthy relationship has no room for physical or emotional abuse. None.

Unfortunately, abuse in relationships is pretty common. According to the Centers for Disease Control and Prevention (CDC), nearly one in four women (22.3 percent) and one in seven men (14.0 percent) age 18 and older have been the victim

of severe physical violence by an intimate partner in their lifetime in the United States.[5]

Abuse can take an enormous toll on anyone. It affects mental
and physical health, work, families, relationships, finances—
essentially all aspects of life. Abusive situations can be complicated. Your partner may be all hearts and flowers at the beginning
of your relationship or their intense attention can seem flattering, but it can gradually emerge that they are manipulative and
controlling. While it can seem logical to cut and run, it can be
difficult to extract yourself from a situation where there is or has
been some good and where you have made a commitment. Abusers are often great at making their partners feel beholden to
them, sometimes by controlling the finances, or their partners
can feel trapped, because after all the abuser's partner has made
a choice and letting the world know they chose an abusive person
would be humiliating. Some abusers are very good at manipulat-
ing the truth and denying things they have said or done. In many
cases, the woman genuinely loves her partner and feels he can
change or believes him when he says he won't abuse her anymore.
Some women stay in a bad situation because they fear angering
their partner and worry about retaliation against them—or their
children, if there are any in the relationship.

RED FLAGS

When you first meet them, abusers can be charming, intense,
and attentive and seem like the greatest thing that ever happened

to you. At first, the need to be with you constantly and that little bit of jealousy can be flattering, but when the intensity is turned up, your partner can turn on you. Warning signs that a partner could potentially become abusive include:[6, 7]

- Constantly texting to see who you are with and what you are doing
- Being very controlling
- Monitoring your social media and phone and demanding access and passwords
- Showing up unexpectedly at work or your home to "check up on you"
- Trying to keep you from your other relationships with friends or family
- Criticizing you in front of others
- Threatening to hurt you or hurt themselves
- Telling you that you are stupid
- Making snide or obnoxious remarks about how you look or how you dress
- Blaming you for their behavior
- Not taking responsibility for their behavior
- Pressuring you for sex
- Seeming "too good to be true"
- Making promises never to do anything to hurt you ever again but failing, repeatedly, to keep that promise

If these red flags emerge, no matter if it is early in the relationship or years into a long-term situation, you need to speak to someone and get some help—a friend; a coworker; a minister, priest, rabbi, or imam; a hotline. It can be difficult to make a break, especially if you care for the person and have been with them for a long time, but it is worth it for your safety. The most important thing to know is that, no matter what your partner says, the abuse is not your fault.

Getting safe and getting help could mean planning ahead to have money stashed or setting up in advance for a safe place to go—a friend or coworker whom your partner doesn't know is a potential option—documenting any injuries/incidents and having duplicates of things like medications or glasses stashed at work or your friend's in case you need to make a quick decision to leave.

EMOTIONAL ABUSE

The pain emotional abuse inflicts is less visible, but it can take a major toll on your self-worth and your psyche. If your partner uses words as weapons and you are the target, you can sometimes feel as if they are justified in what they say—maybe not at first, but as time goes on, their name-calling and blaming can build up, and they can be very convincing that you are flawed and always at fault.

Emotional abuse can be silent, as in your partner giving you the silent treatment or avoiding contact of any kind as punishment for your perceived transgressions. A woman can find herself walking on eggshells so as not to set off her partner or going to great lengths to orchestrate everything—including the way she dresses, talks, or behaves as well as who she spends time with—to prevent her partner from blowing up. It may never get physical, but this sort of behavior is still abusive and toxic.

Everyone gets angry and yells once in a while. If a partner blows up on occasion, it is not necessarily verbal abuse. It's when there is constant yelling that there is a problem. It's the frequency that matters, not the volume. In fact, verbal abuse doesn't have to entail yelling at all or need to be done loudly. It can be as subtle as a whisper powerful enough to undermine your confidence with constant name-calling or threats. Often, people will find themselves in a verbally abusive situation because they were verbally abused in their childhood, even if they may not realize that they were verbally abused, so any shame and criticism heaped on them by a partner feels familiar and possibly deserved—except that it isn't. The legacy can be passed on to children as well. Someone who is verbally abused is prone to suffering from anxiety or depression. The impact of the abuse can be far-reaching into all relationships and work situations—the abuse can make a woman feel as if she is not

---

SEXUAL ASSAULT OR RAPE?

The two terms are often used interchangeably and sometimes *sexual assault* is used in place of the word *rape* to soften the description of what happened. *Sexual assault* is the general term for any unwanted sexual behavior, and *rape* is reserved for forced sexual penetration.

worthy of love, friendships, or success. The good news is that you can get beyond the abuse, learn what a healthy relationship is like, and develop new positive relationships.

Breaking free will take effort as well as support from friends or a women's shelter or therapist. It's not easy—especially if the messages of inadequacy have been internalized—but it can be done.

SEXUAL ASSAULT

The statistics on sexual assault do not paint a pretty picture:

- One in 5 women and 1 in 71 men in the United States have been raped in their lifetime.
- Almost half of female (46.7%) and male (44.9%) victims of rape in the United States were raped by an acquaintance.
- Of these, 45.4% of female rape victims and 29% of male rape victims were raped by an intimate partner.[8]

Do these stats mean that you need to hide away and never go out, never have a drink, never go on a date? No. Locking yourself up in a room isn't the solution. One thing that may help is raising awareness about what sexual assault and rape are, what consent is, what women can do to prevent themselves from being assaulted, and what actions they can take if they are raped or assaulted. Raising awareness can also empower bystanders to give assistance if a woman is in a bad situation.

The consent thing seems pretty easy, right? *No* means *no.*

End of story. But as we've seen from multiple news reports and court cases, it's apparently not that clear-cut. Culturally, we often engage in victim blaming (which not only keeps women from reporting assault but also makes women feel that they somehow caused what happened to them). Questions that come up after an assault are often along these lines: What was she wearing? Was she drunk? Had she been out with him before? What time was it? Did they just meet that night? The big question that isn't often asked is: Why did he assault her? A lot more time seems to be spent on how women can avoid being raped— don't run alone, don't let someone get you a drink, don't leave your drink unattended on the bar—than in teaching people what sexual assault is, what consent is, and telling them not to rape. The truth is that *all* nonconsensual sex is sexual assault. If someone is not able to agree to having sex or is physically forced to have sex or is pressured to have sex or is guilted into having sex—it is not right, and that person is being violated. Not only is it not right, it's illegal. Additionally, if someone stands by, sees a sexual assault, and does nothing, that is not right. Someone who is unconscious cannot consent to sex. Someone who is completely intoxicated cannot consent to sex. If someone says yes to sex on Tuesday, they can say no on Wednesday. If someone is sexually active, it doesn't mean that they want to have sex with anyone and everyone at any time. It's always their choice to say yes or no, and that yes or no needs to be respected. They have the right to change their mind.

Bottom line: If consent is not or cannot be given, it is assault.

The important takeaway here is that consent is a choice that

STEALTH ATTACK

There is a scary form of sexual assault called "stealth-ing," which is nonconsensual condom removal. In other words, you have agreed to use a condom for sex, but he sneakily removes the condom at some point during sex and continues bareback, opening you up to potential risk for STIs or pregnancy.[9] Just because you said yes to sex at first, when he took off that condom, intentionally deceiving you, the act became sexual assault.

---

you make regarding engaging in sexual behavior with someone. If you have not given your consent, then you have been assaulted.

IF YOU HAVE BEEN RAPED OR ASSAULTED

Get to a safe space. A friend. Home. A doctor. A hospital. The police. Resist the urge to change your clothes, shower, or clean yourself, as you may need to have a sexual assault forensic exam, also known as a "rape kit," taken so there is physical and medical evidence of what has happened to you on file, including DNA evidence from your body and clothing. Even if you don't want to report the rape to police or legal authorities or you are unsure, it is a good idea to seek medical attention to assess your health, be sure you are physically okay, discuss any risk for sexually transmitted infections or for pregnancy, and preserve any evidence that might be useful in the future. Call a hotline or a friend for support and try to record as many details as you can remember so that if you do decide to take legal action, you have the incident documented carefully. As difficult as it may be to seek medical care and report the rape to the police, it is very important to do it. Women have said that they felt ashamed and scared after being assaulted, and they wanted nothing more than for it to be over and to not be reminded of it or think about it ever again, but if someone commits assault it is likely they will do it again. Women have also stated that going through the process of reporting the crime can help them move from being a victim to being a survivor.

That being said, the system does not always work in a woman's favor. Rape culture and victim blaming can make it difficult for women to come forward and speak up and take action over what has happened to them. There have been multiple incidents in recent years where a rapist has not been prosecuted to the full extent of the law or that inaction of local law enforcement or, in the case of college campuses, administrations have not been supportive or taken decisive action when a woman has been assaulted. This lack of action certainly can take a toll on a woman who has been raped or attacked and who wants to get help and see that the attacker is found and held responsible for his actions. It can also discourage women from speaking up because they fear they will be blamed, not believed, and will be retraumatized if they have to go through the courts or report the attack to campus administrators.

Many women, following an assault or rape, are fearful of intimacy, being alone, being in a crowd, going near the location of their assault. Many suffer from PTSD (posttraumatic stress

THE RAPE KIT BACKLOG

Unfortunately, lack of funding, lack of time, and lack of resources have left many rape kits untested in storage in police departments and crime labs across the country. This limits the ability of a woman to prosecute an attacker, and it also diminishes the ability of law enforcement to find a repeat offender. An organization called End the Backlog (www.endthebacklog.org) seeks to raise awareness for the issue as well as to promote legislation and policies that will get the kits tested and get the evidence that the kits will provide.

disorder). The stress of the attack can cause anxiety, sleep disorders, or panic attacks, and these can be triggered by being in an intimate situation, seeing someone who looks like the attacker, or being near where the assault took place. Some women turn to alcohol or drugs to numb their feelings or to blot out their intrusive memories of what happened.

Rape or assault takes a devastating toll. But there is help. Multiple hotlines and groups specialize in information and support for women (see Resources). For some women, simply talking about what happened to them helps. With the statistics about assault and rape the way they are, the odds point to a woman finding a friend who has been assaulted or who knows someone who has been assaulted.

Talking about assault and rape and bringing these issues out into the open can help reduce the shame and stigma surrounding sexual assault. And it can help clear the air for conversations about how these assaults can be prevented. It can encourage and support education and discussion about how to keep these incidents from happening. Confiding in someone and finding support can also be extremely helpful in working through the aftermath of the trauma. Healing from any trauma can take time, and a trauma that is so physically and emotionally violating will need ample time and support for healing to take place. Seeking out help is not a sign of weakness; rather, it is a sign that you are strong enough to take the necessary steps to help yourself.

HELPING A FRIEND

If a friend has been raped, help her get the medical attention she needs. Listen, believe, and encourage her to speak with someone—a hotline or support group—but do not force her to do so. Maintain her confidentiality, and don't tell anyone unless she says it is okay. If she wants to report the incident, support her and help her do so, but do not push her if she does not want to make a report. Keep listening. Let her tell you what she needs and when, even if it's hard and her decision is not the one you think that you would make in her place.

INTIMACY AFTER AN ASSAULT

Feeling sexual or deriving pleasure from sex can be challenging if you are a survivor of assault or rape. You may need to relearn how to allow yourself to feel pleasure. One thing you can to is to put yourself in control of how you experience pleasure by masturbating and to allow yourself to feel pleasure from self-love. You can explore safely without any outside pressure or judgment.

If you have been assaulted or raped, then the idea of being intimate with a partner can be difficult. As with all things in relationships, communication can help clear the way to making a healthy connection with your partner and one that feels safe for you. Letting a new partner know that you are a survivor of rape is a first step in being straightforward and clear in the relationship. You may also want to share if there are ways that you do not want to be touched or positions or situations you are going to pass on because they will remind you of your assault. You will heal, but it can take some time for you to feel safe and fulfilled in your sex life.

If you are fortunate enough to never have been bullied, catcalled, abused, or assaulted, there is still much you can do for friends, family, or strangers who have been through the unthinkable. Volunteer, vote, and lend your time and, if possible, your financial support to organizations that give shelter, advice, and assistance to women who need it.

7

YOU AND YOUR V IN THE 21ST C

RELATIVELY SPEAKING, THE VAGINA is not a large part of your anatomy, but having one has a huge influence on your health, your sex life, and your psyche, as well as how you are treated in the world.

The vagina is an amazing little organ. Its diminutive size belies its influence—no matter what anyone says, vaginas really can't become "too loose." It is actually pretty versatile. It allows menstrual blood to exit your body; it is the doorway for sexual intercourse, masturbation, and all forms of sexy play; and it serves as the exit ramp for a baby. That's a lot of jobs for your vag, and *your* job is to keep it well fed with healthy foods and probiotics and to keep it lubed in general as well as when you are having sex.

Having a vagina brings with it benefits and responsibilities. Obviously, it is important to take charge of your health and give your vagina the care and attention it needs. Part of that care is understanding how your vagina is connected to the rest of your body and how protecting your vagina via safer sex and getting regular health screenings can protect you from contracting potentially damaging diseases like HIV/AIDS. A visit to the gyno can catch and treat other diseases, infections, and disorders, including those that are sexually transmitted as well as diseases like cervical cancer. So be sure to get to your gyno on the regular and work with another health professional if you need added guidance on nutrition or for your general and mental health. You should also seek out the care of specialists if you are dealing with a medical condition that could have an impact on your overall or reproductive health (like diabetes, thyroid issues, or an autoimmune disorder).

If tending to vaginal health has benefits for a woman's health as a whole, then we think that the overall health of women can have a positive impact on society as a whole. Without available health care and access to accurate information, women can become unintentionally pregnant, be exposed to sexually transmitted diseases, and miss the opportunity to be screened or treated for everything from cervical cancer to hepatitis. Clinics and affordable health care can allow women to make choices about their bodies and their care that will keep them safe, whole, and healthy. It will allow them to continue contributing to their families, their friendships, their relationships, their employers and employees—doing their part as citizens of their town, state, country, and the world—unimpeded by the mental, emotional, and financial cost of a health issue.

Although *Roe v. Wade* is still the law of the land, there are state legislatures chipping away at a woman's right to choose by curtailing access to birth control, shutting down clinics, and imposing unrealistic "rules" about how, when,[1] and where a woman can seek an abortion. These rules are often made by politicians, not physicians. Inherent in *Roe v. Wade* is the supposition that a woman can choose for herself if she does, or does not, want to have an abortion. Her body; her choice. However, we live in uncertain times, and while we do not want to go back to the days when women put their lives at risk to terminate an unwanted pregnancy, it may seem as if we are heading in that direction.[2] Fortunately, at the moment, taking a pregnancy to term remains a personal choice, and women can determine for themselves if they want to give birth, give a child up for adoption, or end the pregnancy. All options should remain open.

If these rights to birth control, access to medical and prenatal care for women, or abortion are being curtailed in your state, you can protest, vote, and make your voice heard.[3] You can donate your time or money to an organization of your choice that advocates for women's reproductive rights. You can become an escort at a clinic to help women feel safe when they are seeking care.[4]

At the end of the day, affordability and availability of health care can impact women's reproductive health. If insurance does not cover birth control or other services like testing and treatment of sexually transmitted diseases as well as abortion, it leaves women unable to prevent pregnancy or get the care they need. Access to quality care should be every person's right, but unfortunately the reality is very different.

Oddly enough, being a person with a vagina creates a number of paradoxes as you navigate the big bad world. We live in a crazy world where a woman can be harassed as she is walking to her job as CEO of a corporation, being treated like a sexual object and catcalled one minute and then calling the shots in the next. Women in certain fields are subject to "bro culture" that denigrates them and excludes them—we're looking at you, tech and science industries—simply because they are not "bros."

We live in a crazy world where women make 78 cents compared to each dollar their male counterparts take home, often for the same job. Does having a vagina make you less capable of working, learning, leading? We answer with a resounding "No!" There is still work to be done to bridge the gaps not only in opportunities for women but also in the pay gap many women experience. That glass ceiling has many cracks, but it still seems pretty solid in some respects as well.

We live in a world where women have choices and control over how they have sex, but with that freedom can come challenges. With social media, apps, and the general sexual liberation of women, a woman can engage in a new version of "meet market"— as opposed to the "meat markets" of the past when people met at bars and clubs—and find partners for anything from casual hookups to committed relationships with a few swipes on a cell phone. Freedom of choice is awesome, but there are those who will take advantage of a woman looking for a connection and not be honest about themselves or their intentions. We live in a world where we can, through social media, be "friends" with total strangers. Not to put an extra burden on extracurricular activities, but safety first and foremost is important whether you meet via an online app or in line at the DMV.

It's liberating, amazing, and fun to be able to send an intimate photo to a partner to spice up the relationship, and it's devastating when that photo is used for shaming and photographic payback if the relationship doesn't work out. The majority of revenge porn and slut shaming only goes against the people who have vaginas. While we all hear about celebrities who have fallen prey to revenge porn, there have been instances at universities and even in the Marines where women's intimate photos and explicit videos have been shared without their consent as a way of punishing or shaming them. A sex tape is a great way to share intimate moments with your partner—that is, until it is shared with the entire World Wide Web.

Does this mean that women need to become prudish about social media? No, but it does mean that thinking twice before hitting Send or Post is a wise choice and solid advice for everything from e-mail to Twitter to Facebook. If you think that because a site promises that your exchanges will disappear after a few seconds that it's safe to share private images, you can think again, because once a pic is out there, it may stay somewhere forever. Those snaps and posts could come back to haunt you.

As much as women have gained in the world, there is still a lot of shame heaped on women's bodies via everything from advertisers, who airbrush and Photoshop photos into images of unrealistic bodies and send those pics out in the world as paragons of the female form, to porn, where women have flawless bodies devoid of perceived imperfections—including hair—and who give and receive pleasure and multiple orgasms every time with no hangups, no issues, and often with no condoms. Because so many people's first sexual "experience" is actually watching porn, it sets up some impossible expectations for the bedroom and body image for both males and females. Because the first vulva a dude may see is on a screen and there is no hair down there, when he sees a woman's lady parts in IRL he expects the same hair-free space. He can reject and body-shame a woman for something that is completely natural. Expectations and behaviors over sex are often influenced and driven by porn and other media. On the other hand, porn can be a useful tool in figuring out what excites you, give you ideas on how to be more adventurous in the bedroom, and open lines of communication about all things sexual with your partner.

If you have a vagina, then you need to be aware of rape culture and what it is and isn't. Are all males predatory and looking to take advantage of any woman who crosses their paths? No, absolutely not. On the other hand, there seems to be an imbalance of expectations and punishment when it comes to sexual assault and rape. Women are told to keep their knees together or not drink too much at parties or bars. And guys are told, "Boys will be boys." Um, how is this remotely protective of women, and how does it help dudes to understand they have to take responsibility for their actions and be held accountable? We all need to pay attention to what consent is, and what it isn't, and not to turn a blind eye toward behavior that crosses a line.

It has been said that the future is female. Does this mean that all men are going to disappear and women are going to take over the world? Yes. No. Maybe. LOL. Truly, the future is full of possibility for women. But we can't get there if we don't go together and support one another in the quest for education and empowerment in this country and others.

In our time together at Vagina U, we hope you have gained some new perspective on the care and nurturing of your vagina. We've pointed out the health pitfalls you may face that are uniquely female as well as, we hope, given you some new information on how you can express yourself sexually—always safely—and maybe given you some new ideas or inspiration on how to live, love, and learn as a woman with a vagina in the 21st century.

ACKNOWLEDGMENTS

Women need to help each other out with information, support, and even a little inspiration, so I'm happy to have worked with some great women to make this book possible.

The editors of Womenshealthmag.com have been giving women the information they need to navigate with world of women's health, relationships, and more in articles that cover the issues in an accessible and informative way. Thank you, editors, for getting the issues out there and providing such excellent source material for this book.

To Wendy Sherman, thank you for your support and belief that I could get the job done.

To Allison Janice, thanks for your enthusiasm and commitment to this project. You are a true advocate for women!

To everyone at Rodale who helped to dot the I's and cross the Ts, I am grateful for your contribution.

Finally, thank you to my family for their support and understanding.

—Sheila Curry Oakes

RESOURCES

Womenshealthmag.com is a resource and archive for many articles on women's health and well-being. Log on and surf through current and past information on how not only to better understand your body but to get information on how to best take care of your health and well-being.

Following are some links for organizations where you can find further information and support on issues that we have discussed in Vagina U. This is a curated list, so chances are if you have any further questions on an issue that is important to you, it is likely that you will find what you need in one of the sites named here.

HEALTH

Information on health issues from organizations that cover women's and general health.

All-Options (pregnancy info): www.all-options.org
American College of Obstetricians and Gynecologists: www
.acog.org

Centers for Disease Control and Prevention: www.cdc.gov

Get Yourself Tested: www.itsyoursexlife.com/stds-testing-gyt

National Abortion Federation: https://prochoice.org

National Institute of Mental Health: www.nimh.nih.gov

National Women's Health Information Center (NWHIC): www.womenshealth.gov

PERSONAL AND POLITICAL

Organizations that deal with issues related to women's health—in the United States and globally. They are sources of information, inspiration, and activism.

Days for Girls (provides sanitary supplies so girls can go to school): www.daysforgirls.org

Free the Tampons: www.freethetampons.org

GLADD: www.glaad.org

Human Rights Campaign: www.hrc.org

Legalize "Vagina": www.legalizev.com

NARAL Pro-Choice America: www.prochoiceamerica.org

NOW, National Organization for Women: http://now.org

PFLAG: www.pflag.org

Planned Parenthood: www.plannedparenthood.org

Where's the Family Planning?!: www.engenderhealth.org/wtfp

EMERGENCY CONTRACEPTION

Online sources for emergency contraception. Your state and local laws may need to be considered before you order products.

AfterPill: https://afterpill.com

Ella: www.ella-kwikmed.com

RESEARCH

Up-to-date information on research on women's health issues.

The Guttmacher Institute (a primary source of research and policy analysis on abortion, contraception, HIV and STIs, pregnancy, and teens in the United States and internationally): www.guttmacher.org/state-policy/explore/overview-abortion-laws

GENERAL INFORMATION

A source for medical marijuana that is specifically targeted for women's health.

Whoopi & Maya (medical cannabis): http://whoopiandmaya.com

SEXUAL HARASSMENT, ASSAULT, RAPE, ABUSE

Resources and information on reporting rape and assault as well as sources for support and information in workplace and general harassment.

Hollaback! (street harassment, online harassment, gender justice): www.ihollaback.org

It's On Us: www.itsonus.org

Know Your IX: www.knowyourix.org

RAINN (Rape, Abuse & Incest National Network): 1-800-656-HOPE (4673) www.rainn.org

Stop Street Harassment: www.stopstreetharassment.org/2014/06/cardsagainstharassment

US Equal Employment Opportunity Commission: www.eeoc.gov/laws/types/sexual_harassment.cfm

Voices Beyond Assault: www.voicesbeyondassault.org

INTERNET SAFETY

Increase your understanding of how to connect safely in cyberspace.

Cyber Civil Rights Initiative: www.cybercivilrights.org

Cyber Civil Rights Legal Project: www.cyberrightsproject.com

HeartMob: https://iheartmob.org

Stop. Think. Connect.: www.stopthinkconnect.org

Without My Consent: http://withoutmyconsent.org

DOMESTIC VIOLENCE

Where to go for help and information regarding domestic abuse.

Love Is Respect: www.loveisrespect.org

National Coalition Against Domestic Violence: http://ncadv.org

National Domestic Violence Hotline: 1-800-799-7233; www.thehotline.org

National Network to End Domestic Violence: http://nnedv.org

Safe Horizon: www.safehorizon.org

ENDNOTES

CHAPTER 1

1 Koutsky, Judy. "7 Myths about Your Labia That Are Totally Bogus." *Women's Health*. December 29, 2016. http://www.womenshealthmag .com/health/labia-myths/slide/7.

2 Barnes, Zahra. "The Size of Your Vagina: Is It Normal?" *Women's Health*. May 16, 2017. http://www.womenshealthmag.com/health /vagina-size.

3 O'Rourke, Theresa. "Your Private Parts: A Lesson in Female Anatomy." *Women's Health*. May 16, 2017. http://www.womenshealthmag.com /beauty/female-anatomy/page/3/0?utm_content=listiclefooter&utm _medium=Outbrain&utm_source=womenshealthmag.com.

4 Hauser, Christine. "Meet Evatar: The Lab Model That Mimics the Female Reproductive System." *New York Times*. March 30, 2017. https://www.nytimes.com/2017/03/30/science/menstrual-cycle-in-a-dish.html?_r=0

5 Heiser, Christina. "7 Women Speak Up about Why You Shouldn't Be Afraid to Say 'Vagina.'" *Women's Health*. November 1, 2016. http:// www.womenshealthmag.com/health/vagina-campaign.

6 Jacobson, Malia. "How Your Vagina Changes in Your 20s, 30s, and
   40s." *Women's Health*. April 15, 2017. http://www.womenshealthmag
   .com/health/vaginal-changes-with-age.

7 "ACOG Advises against Cosmetic Vaginal Procedures Due to Lack of
   Safety and Efficacy Data." American College of Obstetricians and
   Gynecologists. https://www.acog.org/About-ACOG/News-Room
   /News-Releases/2007/ACOG-Advises-Against-Cosmetic-Vaginal
   -Procedures.

8 Stokes, Rebecca Jane. " 'I Tried the Vagina Shot That's Supposed to
   Make Sex Better—Here's What It Was Like.' " YourTango. November 4,
   2016. http://www.womenshealthmag.com/sex-and-love/what-the-o
   -shot-feels-like.

CHAPTER 2

1 Lusk-Stover, Oni. "Globally, Periods Are Causing Girls to Be Absent
   from School." *Education*. June 27, 2016. http://blogs.worldbank.org/
   education/globally-periods-are-causing-girls-be-absent-school.

2 Hodal, Kate. "Nepal's Bleeding Shame: Menstruating Women
   Banished to Cattle Sheds." *Guardian*. April 1, 2016. https://amp.
   theguardian.com/global-development/2016/apr/01/nepal-bleeding-
   shame-menstruating-women-banished-cattle-sheds.

3 "How to Chart Your Menstrual Cycle." WebMD. February 23, 2016.
   http://www.webmd.com/baby/charting-your-fertility-cycle#1.

4 "The Menstrual Cycle." Womenshealth.gov. January 27, 2017. https://
   www.womenshealth.gov/pregnancy/menstrual-cycle.

5 Dunn, Kyla. "How Do Hormones Work?" PBS. http://www.pbs.org
   /wgbh/pages/frontline/shows/nature/etc/hormones.html.

6 Jacobson, Malia. "5 Hormones That Mess with You Every Month."
   Women's Health. April 15, 2017. http://www.womenshealthmag.com
   /health/female-hormones.

7 Ibid.

8 Utiger, Robert D. "Gonadotropin-Releasing Hormone (GnRH)." *Encyclopædia Britannica*. February 9, 2012. https://www.britannica.com/science/gonadotropin-releasing-hormone.

9 Maron, Dina Fine. "Early Puberty: Causes and Effects." *Scientific American*. May 11, 2015. https://www.scientificamerican.com/article/early-puberty-causes-and-effects/.

10 Ibid..

11 Barnes, Zahra. "7 Reasons You Might Have a Late Period—Other Than Pregnancy." *Women's Health*. August 21, 2017. http://www.womenshealthmag.com/health/late-period.

12 Huhman, Heather. "4 Frustrating Facts about PCOS . . . and What They Mean for You." *Huffington Post*. July 10, 2015. http://www.huffingtonpost.com/heather-huhman/frustrating-facts-about-pcos_b_7686030.html.

13 Kuzma, Cindy. "What Runners Need to Know about Missing Their Periods." *Runner's World*. May 26, 2017. http://www.womenshealthmag.com/fitness/runners-missing-periods.

14 "Do Menstrual Cycles Sync? Unlikely, Finds Clue Data." Hello from Clue. March 9, 2017. http://blog.helloclue.com/post/158185861431/do-menstrual-cycles-sync-unlikely-finds-clue.

15 Walsh, Karla. "7 Period Myths That Need to Go Away Right Now." *Women's Health*. January 11, 2017. http://www.womenshealthmag.com/health/period-myths/slide/1.

16 Devash, Meirav. "3 Moves That Soothe Cramps." *Women's Health*. January 20, 2017. http://www.womenshealthmag.com/fitness/yoga-moves-soothe-cramps.

17 Richards, Sarah Elizabeth. "8 Major Period Problems—Solved." *Women's Health*. April 15, 2017. http://www.womenshealthmag.com/health/period-problems.

18 Brabaw, Kasandra. "8 Facts Every Woman Should Know about Pooping." *Women's Health*. May 18, 2016. http://www.womenshealthmag.com/health/normal-pooping-habits

19 Bender, Rachel. "This Is Why Your Stomach Goes So Crazy during Your Period." Greatist. March 2, 2017. https://greatist.com/grow/digestion-during-period.

20 Edgar, Julie. "Herbal Remedies for PMS." WebMD. November 7, 2015. http://www.webmd.com/women/pms/features/herbal-treatments-for-pms#1.

21 "Herbal Treatments for PMS." Women's Health Network. https://www.womenshealthnetwork.com/pms-and-menstruation/herbal-treatments-for-pms.aspx?utm_source=rss&utm_medium=rss&utm_campaign=herbal-treatments-for-pms.

22 Editors of *Women's Health*. "Premenstrual Syndrome (PMS)." *Women's Health*. March 24, 2016. http://www.womenshealthmag.com/health/premenstrual-syndrome-pms.

23 Daw, Jennifer. "Is PMDD Real?" American Psychological Association. October 2002. http://www.apa.org/monitor/oct02/pmdd.aspx.

24 "Menstruation FAQs." Kotex FAQs. http://www.kotexfits.com/faqs/menstruation/#a3.

25 Olmstead, Susan C. "ACOG: The Menstrual Cycle Is a Vital Sign." *Contemporary OB/GYN*. December 14, 2015. http://contemporaryobgyn.modernmedicine.com/contemporary-obgyn/news/acog-menstrual-cycle-vital-sign.

26 Nunez, Alanna. "6 Things the Color of Your Period Blood Says about Your Health." Women's Health. February 24, 2017. http://www.womenshealthmag.com/health/color-of-your-period-blood-and-health/slide/1.

27 Tommlin, Annie. "Can Sharks Really Smell Your Period Blood?" *Women's Health*. June 22, 2017. http://www.womenshealthmag.com/health/ocean-swimming-myths.

28 Fetters, Ashley. "The Tampon: A History." *Atlantic*. June 1, 2015. https://www.theatlantic.com/health/archive/2015/06/history-of-the-tampon/394334/.

29 Kane, Jessica. "Here's How Much a Woman's Period Will Cost Her over a Lifetime." Huffington Post. May 18, 2015. http://www.huffingtonpost .com/2015/05/18/period-cost-lifetime_n_7258780.html.

30 Fetters, Ashley. "The Tampon: A History." *Atlantic*. June 1, 2015. https://www.theatlantic.com/health/archive/ 2015/06/history-of-the-tampon/394334/.

31 "Toxic Shock Syndrome Bacteria—Topic Overview." WebMD. http:// www.webmd.com/women/tc/toxic-shock-syndrome-bacteria-topic -overview.

32 "Understanding Toxic Shock Syndrome—The Basics." WebMD. http://www.webmd.com/women/guide/understanding-toxic-shock -syndrome-basics#1.

33 Narins, Elizabeth. "This Model Says She Lost Her Leg from Using Tampons." *Cosmopolitan*. July 21, 2017. http://www.cosmopolitan .com/health-fitness/news/a42212/model-lost-leg-from-tampons/.

34 Lanquist, Lindsey. "These Women Tested Out Vintage Period Belts, and It Didn't Go Well." *SELF*. May 25, 2017. https://www.self.com /story/these-women-tested-out-vintage-period-belts-and-it-didnt -go-well.

35 Coughlin, Sara. "The First Menstrual Cup in History Was . . . Complicated." First Menstrual Cup Period Invention History. June 12, 2015. http://www.refinery29.com/2015/06/89096/first -menstrual-cup-history.

36 "Short History of Menstrual Cups." Lunette Menstrual Cup. https:// www.lunette.com/blogs/news/short-history-of-menstrual-cups.

37 "A Brief History of Period Panties." Stuff Mom Never Told You. January 23, 2015. http://www.stuffmomnevertoldyou.com/blogs /a-brief-history-of-period-panties.htm.

38 "Menopause and Perimenopause." *Women's Health*. May 9, 2013. http://www.womenshealthmag.com/health/menopause-and -perimenopause.

39 Weiss, Suzannah. "Federal Prisons Are Finally Giving Women the Dignity of Free Tampons." *Glamour.* August 16, 2017. https://www.glamour.com/story/federal-prisons-women-inmates-free-tampons-pads?utm_content=buffer0a43b&utm_medium=social&utm_source=facebook.com&utm_campaign=buffer.

CHAPTER 3

1 Fetters, Aleisha. "The History of Birth Control." *Women's Health.* May 24, 2010. http://www.womenshealthmag.com/health/history-of-birth-control.
2 "Relative Effectiveness of Birth Control Methods." Options for Sexual Health. March 2009. https://www.optionsforsexualhealth.org/birth-control-pregnancy/birth-control-options/effectiveness.
3 Ryan, Lisa. "We're Finally One Step Closer to Birth Control for Men." The Cut. October 27, 2016. Accessed https://www.thecut.com/2016/10/were-finally-one-step-closer-to-a-male-birth-control-shot.html.
4 "The History of Condoms." LifeStyles. http://www.lifestyles.com/article/the-history-of-condoms/.
5 Nikolchev, Alexandra. "A Brief History of the Birth Control Pill." PBS. May 7, 2010. http://www.pbs.org/wnet/need-to-know/health/a-brief-history-of-the-birth-control-pill/480/.
6 "Menstruation and Menstrual Suppression Survey." Association of Reproductive Health Professionals. http://www.arhp.org/Publications-and-Resources/Studies-and-Surveys/Menstruation-and-Menstrual-Suppression-Survey/fact-sheet.
7 Brady, Krissy. "Exactly What to Do If You Forget to Take Your Birth Control Pill." *Women's Health.* July 25, 2017. http://www.womenshealthmag.com/health/what-to-do-if-you-forget-to-take-your-birth-control-pill?utm_campaign=DailyDose&utm_source

=womenshealthmag.com&utm_ medium=newsletter&smartcode
=YN_0023394221_0001631188&sha1hashlower=406e3a72efa6ce
304ff1bc90cb85659a73ac4066&md5hash=923bbe425ef40a4801b
763b6e105e26a&utm_content=082917.

8 Aggeler, Madeleine. "Do You Really Have to Get Your Period Every
   Month?" Bustle. August 14, 2017. https://www.bustle.com/p/do-you
   -really-have-to-get-your-period-every-month-70471.

9 Carroll, Aaron E. "Birth Control Causes Depression? Not So Fast."
   New York Times. April 3, 2017. https://www.nytimes.com/2017
   /04/03/upshot/birth-control-causes-depression-not-so-fast.html.

10 "Birth Control Pill: Side Effects, Effectiveness, How the Pill Works,
   and Types." WebMD. August 12, 2016. http://www.webmd.com/sex
   /birth-control/birth-control-pills#4-14.

11 Doyle, Kathryn. "Women on Accutane Need Better Contraceptive
   Knowledge." Reuters. February 11, 2015. http://www.reuters.com
   /article/us-health-dermatology-contraception-wome-idUSKBN0LF
   2F420150211.

12 "Best Inventions of 2002." *Time*. November 18, 2002. http://content
   .time.com/time/specials/packages/article/0,28804,1934259_1934672
   _1934717,00.html.

13 "Birth Control Bingo: Depo-Provera." Scarleteen. July 13, 2016.
   http://www.scarleteen.com/birth_control_bingo_depo_provera.

14 "Birth Control Options: The Implant." *Women's Health*. May 6, 2017.
   http://www.womenshealthmag.com/health/birth-control-implant.

15 Schumaker, Erin. "5 Myths about IUDs You Need to Stop Believing."
   Huffington Post. August 25, 2015. http://www.huffingtonpost.com
   /entry/5-myths-about-iuds-you-need-to-stop-believing_us_55d74c
   7fe4b04ae49702f896.

16 Brady, Krissy. "6 Things You Need to Know about Sex When You Have
   an IUD." *Women's Health*. April 4, 2017. http://www.womenshealthmag
   .com/sex-and-love/sex-with-an-iud/slide/1.

17 "How Does the Copper IUD Work as Emergency Contraception?"
    Planned Parenthood. https://www.plannedparenthood.org/learn
    /morning-after-pill-emergency-contraception/how-does-copper-iud
    -work-emergency-contraception.

18 Gomez, Alexandra. "Is Your Birth Control REALLY Making You
    Gain Weight?" *Women's Health*. April 27, 2017. http://www
    .womenshealthmag.com/weight-loss/birth-control-weight-gain.

19 "Birth Control Options: Emergency Contraception." *Women's
    Health*. May 6, 2017. http://www.womenshealthmag.com/health
    /emergency-contraception.

20 Davies, Connor. "The Girl's Guide to Getting Emergency
    Contraception." Bedsider. March 28, 2016. https://www
    .bedsider.org/features/363-the-girl-s-guide-to-getting-emergency
    -contraception).

21 Rodriguez, Maria Isabel, MD. "5 Myths about the Emergency
    Contraceptive Pill, Busted." Bedsider. February 21, 2017. https://
    www.bedsider.org/features/232-5-myths-about-the-emergency
    -contraceptive-pill-busted.

22 Pollitt, Katha. "Abortion in American History." *Atlantic*. August 10,
    2017. https://www.theatlantic.com/magazine/archive/1997/05
    /abortion-in-american-history/376851/.

23 Walsh, Karla. "Everything You Need to Know about the Abortion
    Pill." *Women's Health*. May 6, 2017. http://www.womenshealthmag
    .com/health/abortion-pill.

24 Reagan, Leslie J. *When Abortion Was a Crime: Women, Medicine, and
    Law in the United States, 1867–1973*. Berkeley, CA: University of
    California Press, 2008.

25 Pollitt, Katha. "Abortion in American History." *Atlantic*. August 10,
    2017. https://www.theatlantic.com/magazine/archive/1997/05
    /abortion-in-american-history/376851/.

26 "Reproductive Health Data and Statistics." Centers for Disease

Control and Prevention. May 10, 2017. https://www.cdc.gov
/reproductivehealth/data_stats/index.htm.

27 "What Happens to Your Vagina during Pregnancy." Ava Women.
https://www.avawomen.com/avaworld/happens-vagina-pregnancy/.

28 "Caesarean Section." *Women's Health*. May 9, 2013. http://www
.womenshealthmag.com/health/caesarean-section.

29 Thielking, Megan. "Why the C-section Rate Is Much Higher Than It
Should Be in US." STAT. March 9, 2016.. https://www.statnews
.com/2015/12/01/cesarean-section-childbirth/.

30 Mayo Clinic Staff. "Sex after Pregnancy: Set Your Own Timeline."
Mayo Clinic. July 2, 2015. http://www.mayoclinic.org/healthy
-lifestyle/labor-and-delivery/in-depth/sex-after-pregnancy/art
-20045669).

31 Mayo Clinic Staff. "Postpartum Depression: Manage Your
Symptoms, Enjoy Your Baby." Mayo Clinic. August 11, 2015. http://
www.mayoclinic.org/diseases-conditions/postpartum-depression
/basics/symptoms/con-20029130.

CHAPTER 4

1 Baldwin, Debby Herbenick, PhD. "What Each of Facebook's 51 New
Gender Options Means." Daily Beast. February 15, 2014. http://www
.thedailybeast.com/what-each-of-facebooks-51-new-gender-options
-means.

2 Ibid.

3 "Sexual Orientation." WebMD. November 8, 2016. http://www.webmd
.com/sex-relationships/guide/sexual-orientation#1).

4 Corinna, Heather. "Sexuality: WTF Is It, Anyway?" Scarleteen. May
10, 2016. http://www.scarleteen.com/article/bodies/sexuality_wtf
_is_it_anyway.

5 Thottam, Isabel. "10 Online Dating Statistics You Should Know

(U.S.)." 10 Online Dating Statistics (for U.S.) You Should Know | eHarmony. https://www.eharmony.com/online-dating-statistics/.

6 Dineen, Cari. "Safe Sex: Lay Down Some Rubber!" *Women's Health*. May 9, 2013. http://www.womenshealthmag.com/sex-and-love/sex-protection.

7 Barnett, Emma. "Female Masturbation i=Isn't Shameful—Here's the Video to Prove It." *Telegraph*. April 14, 2016. http://www.telegraph.co.uk/women/sex/female-masturbation-isnt-shameful---heres-the-video-to-prove-it/.

8 Stampler, Laura. "Here's Why You Should Always Masturbate on Your Period." *Women's Health*. May 16, 2017. http://www.womenshealthmag.com/health/period-masturbation.

9 Barnes, Zahra. "How Likely Are You to Poop During Anal Sex?" *Women's Health*. June 26, 2017. http://www.womenshealthmag.com/sex-and-love/poop-during-anal-sex.

10 Editors of *Women's Health*. "Your Complete Guide to Keeping Your Butthole Healthy." *Women's Health*. April 6, 2017. http://www.womenshealthmag.com/health/butthole-health.

11 Editors of *Women's Health*. "Your Ultimate Guide to Anal Sex." *Women's Health*. August 29, 2017. http://www.womenshealthmag.com/sex-and-love/anal-sex-101.

12 Barnes, Zahra. "What to Do if You Hate the Way His Semen Tastes." *Women's Health*. June 4, 2015. http://www.womenshealthmag.com/sex-and-love/changing-taste-of-semen.

13 Heiser, Christina. "You Need to Share This Video about Hymens with Every Man in Your Life." *Women's Health*. December 9, 2015. http://www.womenshealthmag.com/health/hymen-video

14 Daly, Annie. "Does Your Vagina Become Tighter If You Have Less Sex?" *Women's Health*. April 3, 2015. http://www.womenshealthmag.com/sex-and-love/do-vaginas-get-tighter-with-less-sex.

15 McGuire, Judy. "Here's What Happens to Your Vagina during a

Dry Spell." *Women's Health.* November 4, 2016. http://www
.womenshealthmag.com/sex-and-love/what-happens-to-vagina
-when-you-stop-having-sex.

16 Hrustic, Alisa. "Here's Why Millennials Love These 3 Sex Positions."
Women's Health. May 2, 2017. http://www.womenshealthmag.com
/sex-and-love/millenials-favorite-sex-positions.

17 Beland, Nicole. "The Female Orgasm: How It Works." *Women's Health.*
April 17, 2017. http://www.womenshealthmag.com/sex-and-love/sex
-ed-anatomy-of-an-orgasm.

18 "The World's Weirdest Orgasms." *Women's Health.* April 17, 2017.
http://www.womenshealthmag.com/sex-and-love/different-orgasm.

19 Monaghan, Sheila, Brittany Risher, and Caitlin Carlson. "Your Brain
on an Orgasm." *Women's Health.* April 17, 2017. http://www
.womenshealthmag.com/sex-and-love/orgasm-body.

20 Frederick, David A., H. Kate St. John, Justin R. Garcia, and Elisabeth A.
Lloyd. "Differences in Orgasm Frequency Among Gay, Lesbian,
Bisexual, and Heterosexual Men and Women in a U.S. National Sample."
Archives of Sexual Behavior, 2017. doi:10.1007/s10508-017-0939-z.

21 Crain, Esther. "Consider Yourself Very Lucky if You Don't Have One
of These 5 Vaginal Disorders." *Women's Health.* April 15, 2017. http://
www.womenshealthmag.com/health/vaginal-disorders.

22 "American College of Obstetricians and Gynecologists FAQ:
Endometriosis." American College of Obstetricians and
Gynecologists. October 2012. https://www.acog.org/Patients/FAQs
/Endometriosis.

23 Bratskeir, Kate. "10 Celebs Open Up about Their Struggles with
Endometriosis." Huffington Post. March 15, 2016. http://www
.huffingtonpost.com/entry/celebrities-with-endometriosis_us
_56e1ba4ee4b065e2e3d51bca.

24 Sollee, Kristen. "9 Crazy Sex Myths—Busted!" *Women's Health.*
August 28, 2014. http://www.womenshealthmag.com/sex-and-love
/sex-myths-debunked.

25 Breene, Sophia. "Superfood or Supergross? The Truth about Semen." Greatist. June 6, 2016. https://greatist.com/health/nutrition-of-semen.

26 Benjamin, Jennifer. "Is Your Libido MIA?" *Women's Health*. August 8, 2012. http://www.womenshealthmag.com/life/sex-drive.

27 Booth, Stephanie. "The 6 Biggest Mistakes Couples Make in the Bedroom." *Women's Health*. August 17, 2017. http://www.womenshealthmag.com/sex-and-love/mistakes-couples-make-in-the-bedroom.

28 Folgia, Michelle. "30 Sex Fantasies to Turn into Reality." YourTango. February 14, 2014. http://www.womenshealthmag.com/sex-and-love/sex-fantasies.

29 Castleman, Michael. "A Loving Introduction to BDSM." *Psychology Today*. June 15, 2012. https://www.psychologytoday.com/blog/all-about-sex/201206/loving-introduction-bdsm.

30 DeBellefonds, Colleen. "7 Sexologist-Approved Sex Toys under $20." *Women's Health*. July 19, 2017. http://www.womenshealthmag.com/sex-and-love/amazon-sex-toys-under-20-dollars

31 Miller, Korin. "7 Things You Should Never Use As Lube." *Women's Health*. March 23, 2017. http://www.womenshealthmag.com/sex-and-love/substitute-for-lube/slide/5.

CHAPTER 5

1 Hergenrader, Jamie. "What Does Planned Parenthood DO Exactly?" *Women's Health*. June 9, 2017. http://www.womenshealthmag.com/life/defunding-planned-parenthood.

2 Mendez, Bianca. "Why Are Women Booking Appointments for Professional Vagina Massages?" *Women's Health*. April 15, 2017. http://www.womenshealthmag.com/sex-and-love/yoni-massage.

3 Bruning, Sarah. "Douching Could Double Your Risk for This Type of Cancer." *Women's Health*. April 15, 2017. http://www.womenshealthmag.com/health/douching-ovarian-cancer.

4   Crain, Esther. "Decoding Your Vaginal Discharge." *Women's Health*. April 15, 2017. http://www.womenshealthmag.com/health/vaginal -discharge.

5   "Vaginal Discharge: What's Abnormal?" WebMD. September 18, 2016. http://www.webmd.com/women/guide/vaginal-discharge -whats-abnormal#1.

6   "Vaccines and Preventable Diseases." Centers for Disease Control and Prevention. November 22, 2016. https://www.cdc.gov/vaccines /vpd/hpv/hcp/safety-effectiveness.html.

7   Heiser, Christina. "New Statistics Prove the HPV Vaccine Is Actually Working." *Women's Health*. April 15, 2017. http://www .womenshealthmag.com/health/hpv-vaccine-success.

8   Thomason, Kristine. "Everything You Think You Know about Herpes Is Wrong." Health.com. http://www.health.com/sexual -health/everything-you-think-you-know-about-herpes-is-wrong.

9   "HIV/AIDS." *Women's Health*. May 9, 2013. http://www .womenshealthmag.com/health/hivaids.

10 "Vaccines and Preventable Diseases." Centers for Disease Control and Prevention. November 22, 2016. https://www.cdc.gov/vaccines /vpd/hpv/hcp/safety-effectiveness.html.

11 Heiser, Christina. "New Statistics Prove the HPV Vaccine Is Actually Working." *Women's Health*. April 15, 2017. http://www .womenshealthmag.com/health/hpv-vaccine-success.

12 Brady, Krissy. " 'Yes, That's Acne on Your Vagina—Here's How to Treat It.' " *Women's Health*. June 30, 2017. http://www.womenshealthmag .com/health/vaginal-acne-treatment.

13 Sinrich, Jenn. "What's That on Your Hoo-Ha? 5 Vaginal Conditions You Need to Know About." *Women's Health*. May 19, 2017. http:// www.womenshealthmag.com/health/vaginal-sores-and-bumps-to -know/slide/5.

14 Shortsleeve, Cassie. "8 Reasons for Blood in Your Panties (Other Than Your Period)." *Women's Health*. August 9, 2016. http://www

.womenshealthmag.com/health/random-vaginal-bleeding.

15 Sinrich, Jenn. "What's That on Your Hoo-Ha? 5 Vaginal Conditions You Need to Know About." *Women's Health*. May 19, 2017. http://www.womenshealthmag.com/health/vaginal-sores-and-bumps-to-know/slide/5.

16 Shortsleeve, Cassie. "5 Skin Conditions You Can Get on Your Vagina." *Women's Health*. June 7, 2016. http://www.womenshealthmag.com/health/skin-conditions-on-vagina.

17 "Bladder Infection (Cystitis)." *Women's Health*. May 9, 2013. http://www.womenshealthmag.com/health/bladder-infection-cystitis. Medical content reviewed by the Faculty of the Harvard Medical School. Copyright by Harvard University. All rights reserved. Used with permission of StayWell.

18 Crain, Esther. "5 Reasons Your Vagina Is Going Dry." *Women's Health*. April 15, 2017. http://www.womenshealthmag.com/health/vaginal-dryness.

19 Shortsleeve, Cassie. "5 Skin Conditions You Can Get on Your Vagina." *Women's Health*. June 7, 2016. http://www.womenshealthmag.com/health/skin-conditions-on-vagina.

20 Kloss, Kelsey. "This Is Why Your Vagina Is So Itchy—And How to Make It Stop." *Women's Health*. August 3, 2017. http://www.womenshealthmag.com/health/5-common-reasons-for-vaginal-itching.

21 Shortsleeve, Cassie. "PSA: You Can Bruise, Cut, and Tear Your Vagina." *Women's Health*. August 22, 2016. http://www.womenshealthmag.com/health/vagina-injuries.

22 Mackenzie, Macaela. "Here's How to Prevent Ingrown Pubes Once and For All." *Women's Health*. April 21, 2017. http://www.womenshealthmag.com/beauty/ingrown-pubic-hair.

23 Crain, Esther. "Consider Yourself Very Lucky if You Don't Have One of These 5 Vaginal Disorders." *Women's Health*. April 15, 2017. http://www.womenshealthmag.com/health/vaginal-disorders.

24 Shortsleeve, Cassie. "Must-Know Facts about the Most Common

Cause of Stinky Hoo-Ha." *Women's Health*. December 3, 2015. http://
www.womenshealthmag.com/health/bacterial-vaginosis.

25 Middleton, Tracy. "5 Types of Vaginal Odors You Should Know
about—And What They Mean for Your Health." *Women's Health*. July
24, 2017. http://www.womenshealthmag.com/health/what-your
-vaginal-odor-means.

26 Sinrich, Jenn. "What's That on Your Hoo-Ha? 5 Vaginal Conditions
You Need to Know About." *Women's Health*. May 19, 2017. http://
www.womenshealthmag.com/health/vaginal-sores-and-bumps-to
-know/slide/5.

27 White, Rachel Marie. "How to Get Rid of a UTI Fast, Using Natural
Remedies." Mindbodygreen. July 13, 2017. https://www
.mindbodygreen.com/articles/natural-urinary-tract-infection
-treatments?utm_term=pos-1&utm_source=mbg&utm_medium
=email&utm_content=daily1&utm_campaign=170713.

28 Katsipoutis, Stella. "6 Things You Should NEVER Do When You
Have a UTI." *Women's Health*. August 23, 2017. http://www
.womenshealthmag.com/health/urinary-tract-infections-what-not
-to-do/.

29 Brady, Krissy. "5 Ways to Fight Off UTIs—Or Soothe Symptoms if
You've Already Got One." *Women's Health*. April 13, 2017. http://
www.womenshealthmag.com/health/uti-prevention-methods.

30 White, Rachel. "How to Prevent a UTI." *Women's Health*. November
21, 2012. http://www.womenshealthmag.com/health/how-to
-prevent-a-uti.

CHAPTER 6

1 Miller, Korin. "Scientists Prove That 'Resting Bitch Face' Is a Real
Thing." *Women's Health*. February 3, 2016. http://www
.womenshealthmag.com/life/resting-bitch-face.

2   WITW staff. "Global Study Shows Vast Majority of Women Are Catcalled before the Age of 17." *New York Times*. May 29, 2015. http://nytlive.nytimes.com/womenintheworld/2015/05/29/global-study-shows-vast-majority-of-women-are-catcalled-before-the-age-of-17/.

3   Piercy, Naomi. "How to Handle Sexual Harassment." *Women's Health*. March 3, 2015. http://www.womenshealthmag.com/life/how-to-handle-sexual-harassment.

4   Chokshi, Niraj. "How to Fight Back Against Revenge Porn." *New York Times*. May 18, 2017. https://www.nytimes.com/2017/05/18/us/fighting-revenge-porn.html?_r=0.

5   "Violence Prevention." Centers for Disease Control and Prevention. August 22, 2017. https://www.cdc.gov/violenceprevention/intimatepartnerviolence/consequences.html.

6   Piercy, Naomi. "How to Recognize If You're in an Abusive Relationship." *Women's Health*. November 26, 2012. http://www.womenshealthmag.com/health/how-to-recognize-if-youre-in-an-abusive-relationship.

7   "Red Flags of Abuse." National Network to End Domestic Violence. http://nnedv.org/resources/stats/gethelp/redflagsofabuse.html.

8   "Statistics: National Coalition Against Domestic Violence." NCADV. http://ncadv.org/learn-more/statistics.

9   Hall, Alena. "What You Need to Know about the Disturbing Sexual Assault Trend Called 'Stealthing.'" *Women's Health*. April 24, 2017. http://www.womenshealthmag.com/life/condoms-stealthing-study.

CHAPTER 7

1   Stampler, Laura. "How Late Can You Get an Abortion?" *Women's Health*. August 1, 2017. http://www.womenshealthmag.com/health/how-late-can-you-get-an-abortion.

2   Marty, Robin. "This Is What a Future without Legal Abortions

Would Look Like." *Women's Health*. August 10, 2016. http://www
.womenshealthmag.com/life/what-if-abortion-completely-illegal.

3 Sifferliln, Alexandra. "Donald Trump: States Fighting to Protect
Reproductive Rights." *Time*. February 8, 2017. http://time.com
/4663777/states-protect-reproductive-rights/.

4 Mackenzie, Macaela. "6 Things You Can Do Right Now to Protect
Your Reproductive Rights." *Women's Health*. November 11, 2016.
http://www.womenshealthmag.com/life/protect-female-reproductive
-rights.

INDEX

genital warts/HPV and, 206, 210
itching from, 148
lubricants and, 172, 173, 174
myths about, 80–81, 155
nonconsensual removal of, 245
oral sex and, 137
period sex and, 154
for safer sex, 79–80, 81, 129, 133, 203, 205, 208, 209
sex toys and, 170, 171, 222
syphilis and, 211
types of, 80, 155
for vaginal pH balance, 186
Contact dermatitis, 215–16
Contraception. *See* Birth control methods
Cortisol, 31, 157
Cowgirl sex position, 142, **142**, 153
Crabs, pubic, 210
Cramps, menstrual, 43–46, 132
Cranberry juice, for UTI relief, 224
Cravings, during period, 46–47, 52
Crura, **5**
C-section, 114
Cunnilingus, 82. *See also* Oral sex
Cystitis, 216–17
Cysts
Bartholin's, 214
ovarian, 38, 39, 149–50

D

D&C/D&E, for abortion, 110–11
Dating
online, 125–28, 254–55
in workplace, 231
Dental dams, 82, **82**, 137, 205
Depilatories, for pubic-hair removal, 196
Depo-Provera, 92–94, 93
Depression, postpartum, 116
Dermatitis, contact, 215–16
Diaphragm, 98–100, **98**
Discharge, vaginal, 112, 199–204, 205
D-mannose supplements, for UTI relief, 223
Doggy style sex position, 142–43, **142**

Douching, 50–51, 191, 202
Dryness, vaginal, 19, 74, 147, 149, 217
Dyspareunia, 152

E

Eczema, 217–18, 220
Ejaculate, female, 134–35
Electrolysis, for pubic-hair removal, 197
Emergency contraception, 97, 102–4, 104–105, 108
Emotional abuse, 241–43
Emotional upheaval, during period, 46
Endocrine system, 29
Endometriosis, 9–10, 88, 149–50, 152, 218
Endometrium, 9–10
Endorphins, 147
Episiotomy, 115
Estradiol, 29–30
Estrogen
anorexia and, 36
in birth control pills, 83, 99
early puberty and, 34
functions of, 10, 29–30
in menstrual cycle, 27, 47, 57
"mini pill" without, 85
Exercise
for menstrual cramp relief, 43, 44–45
missed period from, 36
Extended-cycle birth control pills, 86–87

F

Fallopian tubes, **6**, 9, 10, 27
Fantasies, sexual, 162–63
Female athlete triad, missed period from, 37, 39
Female condoms, 81–82, **81**, 205
Female ejaculate, 134–35
Feminine hygiene products, 59–71
Feminine wipes, 137, 190–91
Fertility
emergency contraception and, 105
endometriosis affecting, 150